COPING WITH CANCER IN EARLY ADULTHOOD

Support and Guidance for Patients Ages 18-'49

From Diagnosis to Treatment to Day-to-Day Life Changes, Navigating Your Cancer Journey

CRISTINA POZO-KADERMAN, PhD, and SAUL WISNIA

Foreword by **William F. Pirl, MD, MPH,** *Chair of Psychiatry & Behavioral Sciences at Memorial Sloan Kettering Cancer Center*

ADAMS MEDIA

NEW YORK AMSTERDAM/ANTWERP LONDON TORONTO
SYDNEY/MELBOURNE NEW DELHI

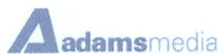

Aadamsmedia

Adams Media
An Imprint of Simon & Schuster, LLC
100 Technology Center Drive
Stoughton, MA 02072

First Adams Media trade paperback edition October 2025

For information about special discounts for bulk purchases, please contact Simon & Schuster Special Sales at 1-866-506-1949 or business@simonandschuster.com.

The Simon & Schuster Speakers Bureau can bring authors to your live event. For more information or to book an event, contact the Simon & Schuster Speakers Bureau at 1-866-248-3049 or visit our website at www.simonspeakers.com.

Manufactured in the United States of America

1 2025

Library of Congress Control Number: 2025940327

ISBN 978-1-5072-2420-5
ISBN 978-1-5072-2421-2 (ebook)

Praise for *Coping with Cancer in Early Adulthood*

"*Coping with Cancer in Early Adulthood* is a heartfelt, easy-to-understand, practical gem filled with useful tips on seeking appropriate and developmentally sensitive cancer care. Young adults no longer have to go on their cancer journey alone. With myth-busting straight talk from Dr. Pozo-Kaderman, an experienced psychologist, young patients with cancer will feel validated that there is 'no right way to feel' about such a devastating diagnosis just at the moment when their personal identities are getting established. This book is a must-have in the office of every oncologist who treats young adults!"
—**Maryland Pao, MD,** Past President of the Academy of Consultation-Liaison Psychiatry and Clinical Professor of Psychiatry at Georgetown University School of Medicine, Washington, DC

"*Coping with Cancer in Early Adulthood* is a must-read for every young adult who is dealing with the existential challenge of cancer. Dr. Pozo-Kaderman has taken her decades of experience and expertise as a psychologist working with adolescents and young adults with cancer to create a comprehensive, thoughtful, and accessible resource for the growing number of young adults in the United States who are being diagnosed and treated for cancer. This book is extremely timely and an essential resource."
—**William Breitbart, MD,** Chairman and Jimmie C. Holland Chair in Psychiatric Oncology, Department of Psychiatry & Behavioral Sciences at Memorial Sloan Kettering Cancer Center

"As an oncologist, I've seen firsthand the unique and significant challenges faced by young adults with cancer. This indispensable guidebook offers comprehensive insights and guidance that are crucial for patients navigating both treatment and survivorship."
—**Ann S. LaCasce, MD, MMSc,** Director of the Dana-Farber/Mass General Brigham Fellowship in Hematology/Oncology and Associate Professor of Medicine at Harvard Medical School

Praise for *Coping with Cancer in Early Adulthood*

"This book is a remarkable compilation of wisdom acquired through years of Dr. Pozo-Kaderman's focused commitment—and hours of listening—to the concerns of young adults with cancer. The style is so approachable, it reads like an extended conversation with Dr. Pozo-Kaderman. This book steps through the many stages of cancer treatment, anticipating the issues and questions likely to arise. I anticipate this book will be helpful not just to young adults but also to the cancer care teams dedicated to helping them."

—**Lindsay Frazier, MD,** Dana-Farber Cancer Institute Physician and Professor of Pediatrics at Harvard Medical School

"Dr. Pozo-Kaderman has distilled decades of professional experience and wisdom into this thoughtful guide for young adult cancer patients. This book provides practical and hopeful guidance and should become an instant classic for newly diagnosed patients, their caregivers, and loved ones."

—**Krishna Komanduri, MD,** Chief, UCSF Health Division of Hematology-Oncology and Julius R. Krevans Distinguished Professor of Medicine at the University of California San Francisco

Contents

Acknowledgments   7

Foreword.   9

Introduction   11

Chapter 1: What's So Different about Cancer
              in Young Adults?   15

Chapter 2: Early Days   31

Chapter 3: Sharing the News and Next Steps   53

Chapter 4: Coping with Cancer Treatment   69

Chapter 5: Emotional and Life Changes.   99

Chapter 6: Well-Being, Mental Health,
              and Self-Care. 125

Chapter 7: Psychotherapy As Part of Treatment . . 149

Chapter 8: Post-Treatment Life. 171

Chapter 9: Sexual Health 193

Chapter 10: Living with Chronic Cancer 213

Conclusion: Living with Purpose 235

Bibliography 237

Resources 245

Index 251

Acknowledgments

This book is dedicated to all the patients and families who have allowed me into their lives. Thank you for teaching me so much. My mom is the inspiration for my work and this book. She taught me what it means to be resilient and to find gratitude even in the most unbearable circumstances. My father and brother have provided infinite support and love throughout my life. Thank you both.

Professionally, I have been extremely fortunate to have worked with and be mentored by the most brilliant, creative, and kind human beings including Frank Miller, Paul Jacobsen, Bill Redd, Bill Breitbart, Steve Passik, Pat Saab, Maryland Pao, Deane Wolcott, Jimmie Holland—the founder of psycho-oncology—and, of course, Bill Pirl, whose faith and encouragement got me to work on this book. Thank you for allowing me to flourish at this stage of my career.

In recent years I have dealt with major losses, and Sue Morris's guidance and friendship have been invaluable. Thanks also to: Karen Fasciano for being so open, welcoming and trusting me with the Young Adult Program (YAP) at Dana-Farber. The entire YAP team, including Joan Hanania, Paige Malinowski, Annelise Ryan, Meghan Donovan, Katelyn Williams, and most importantly, Sarah Fay. The Stone Family for making YAP a reality and allowing young adults with cancer to have access to such needed services. Saul Wisnia, the best writing partner ever. Lizette Benitez, who has been my rock since we were kids. You are the sister I always wanted. My puppies, starting with Salchicha—who taught me the love of dogs—along with Choriza/Choo Choo, Foxy, Havanita, Zoe, and Azalea. Rick, the love of my life, thank you for your unwavering support throughout our marriage. Your patience and understanding are boundless. And to the linchpin of our family, my beloved daughter, Ely. She gives my life meaning and joy. I feel so proud and honored to be your mother.

—CPK

First off, thank you to Dr. Cristina Pozo-Kaderman for allowing me to help bring her incredible knowledge and passion to life in these pages. I know readers will benefit greatly from her insights, as well as those of her patients—whose experiences and reflections can be found throughout the book.

I've spent more than twenty-five years chronicling the lives of cancer patients of all ages at Dana-Farber, including far too many young adults. My thanks to them all for sharing their journeys with me. I am inspired each day by their resilience, just as I am inspired by my home team of Michelle, Jason, and Rachel. They bring me happiness beyond measure, as does Phoebe—my ball hound and running companion.

—SW

Thank you to the entire team at Adams Media and Simon & Schuster, especially editors Laura Daly and Colleen Mulhern. It was Colleen's own experience as a young adult with cancer that served as the genesis for this book, and she and Laura were its champions each step of the way. We appreciate your confidence, support, and excellence.

—CPK and SW

Foreword

By William F. Pirl, MD, MPH

No one ever wants to hear they have cancer. But learning you have cancer as a young adult is especially jarring. Cancer complicates life—and life is already complicated.

While cancer treatments have had remarkable advancements over the last several years, our understanding of how to help people live their lives with cancer has also advanced. Research has shown that when people know what to expect, they actually have better experiences. Being informed can help you make the best choices, manage common side effects, and do the things you need to do in order to have the best possible outcomes.

However, information is also complicated, especially now, with a world of unfiltered material so easily available. Quick searches can result in despair after seeing something you can't unsee and which might not even be related to your cancer. We are also flooded with health influencers who claim cancer can be cured with a smoothie, and conspiracy theories about why your doctor doesn't want you to know about some healing fruit from the Amazon. It also seems like almost everyone knows someone who did something that made their cancer go away; they feel the need to tell you that whatever you are doing is wrong. It can be difficult, even for medical professionals, to sort through all this information coming from every direction.

One of the things people with cancer need to do is figure out an information strategy that works for them: a strategy in which they can get all the benefits of being informed, block out the noise, and not be overwhelmed with information overload. The foundation of this strategy should be your oncology team. Your oncology team can help you interpret any information you have encountered and let you know if it is relevant to you and your specific cancer situation.

I wish every young person with cancer had access to an expert like Dr. Pozo-Kaderman. Dr. Pozo-Kaderman has devoted her entire career as a psychologist to helping people cope with cancer. She leads a program specifically for young adults with cancer at Dana-Farber Cancer Institute. This book shares her knowledge and experience to make what can be an overwhelming situation more manageable. It assembles the essential information needed for young adults to live life with cancer, and it can serve as a trusted resource in your information strategy.

Introduction

"How could this happen to me? I'm so young." "Am I going to die?"
"How could my life change so abruptly in a second?" "How could
this have been growing inside my body without my knowledge?"
"What now?"

No matter your age, hearing the words "You have cancer" is a life-altering moment. For most people, it is impossible to comprehend anything said after those three words. You are flooded with emotions and a sense of unreality, and in that instant begin to ask yourself unanswerable questions. Your life is now divided into two halves—before and after diagnosis—accompanied by overwhelming feelings that may include terror, anger, and sadness.

Unfortunately, these days, more and more young adults like you are finding themselves in this situation. Despite overall improvements in care and survivorship, one trend has become apparent: According to the American Cancer Society (ACS), while cancer incidence has been in general decline during the past decade, the number of young adults with cancer—otherwise known as those with early onset cancer—has increased. I've observed this development firsthand in my more than thirty years as a clinical psychologist specializing in the treatment of cancer patients and their families. I am currently a senior psychologist and director of the Young Adult Program at Dana-Farber Cancer Institute, as well as a faculty member at Harvard Medical School. My coauthor, Saul Wisnia, has spent more than twenty-five years chronicling the experiences of cancer patients—a growing number of them young adults—as senior publications editor-writer at Dana-Farber.

What we've learned through our work is that your experience as a young adult with cancer is unlike that of children or older adults. Despite the fact that more young adults are being diagnosed with cancer than ever before, you have been all but forgotten when it comes to tailored guidance. Pediatric oncology patients (typically those eighteen and younger) receive their care in brightly colored clinics filled with toys and computer games to distract them and special programs to help their parents, siblings, and classmates better cope with and understand their diagnoses. Adults in their fifties, sixties, and beyond (who make up the largest share of the cancer patient population) are surrounded—at treatment, and often within their circles of friends—by peers going through similar experiences. There is no shortage of people ready to offer tips for dealing with side effects, rides to the clinic, or home-cooked meals after long days of chemotherapy.

As a young adult, on the other hand, you endure the shock of a cancer diagnosis and months or even years of treatment without the luxury of a large, supportive group of knowledgeable peers. Your friends, classmates, and colleagues can't relate to what you are going through, and are often too busy dealing with their own lives at work, school, and home to lend much of a hand. Your parents will usually offer everything they can, including your childhood bedroom, but years (or decades) after living away, thoughts of returning to the nest can seem like another step backward when you are already feeling derailed from life. Many young adults may not trust doctors, who often initially misdiagnose or fail to investigate symptoms that could indicate cancer due to their lack of training or experience in treating young adults, among other possible reasons.

Coping with Cancer in Early Adulthood aims to finally speak to you—to give you the specific information, targeted support, and unique guidance you need to face this difficult situation. You'll find advice on how to:

- Deal with a new diagnosis
- Assemble the best treatment team

- Manage social isolation and well-meaning, but toxic, positivity
- Consider often-ignored but vital topics like fertility and sexual health
- Navigate the wide range of emotions that come at different stages of your cancer journey
- Understand common treatments, along with strategies to help manage side effects
- Handle treatment-related interruptions that can leave you feeling out of sync with your peers
- Move forward post-treatment to build a "new normal" at school, at work, and with your family, friends, and life partners
- Face fears of cancer recurrence

Along the way, you'll hear from patients who have been where you are now. Their stories capture a diverse range of life situations and emotional reactions—but most important, they'll show you that you're not alone.

Wherever you are in your journey, *Coping with Cancer in Early Adulthood* can help you manage cancer's emotional and physical toll and explore who you are post-diagnosis. This book will equip you with important information, but also suggest ways to ask others for meaningful support. It will help you find ways to cope and also remind you to be gentle with yourself. You may not be able to change the hand you've been dealt, but you can empower yourself to navigate cancer with knowledge and self-compassion.

—Cristina Pozo-Kaderman, PhD

Keep in mind that you can use this book however works best for you. You could read it from start to finish, or jump right to sections that address a specific situation you need help with at the moment. Feel free to linger longer on topics where you need extra support. Since we're discussing very sensitive subjects, some sections might feel especially painful to read. If that happens, take a break if necessary, skip the section and return to it later, or discuss it with someone on your care team.

CHAPTER 1

What's So Different about Cancer in Young Adults?

Everything seemed to be coming together for Daniella. Ten years out of law school, she was living in a new city she loved and working for a firm focused on labor law—her specialty. She joined a gym, began dating a new guy, and was starting to make friends.

When Daniella developed a cough and began feeling more fatigued than normal, she figured the cause might be allergies related to all the pollen in the early spring air. Only after the symptoms persisted for six weeks did Daniella finally go to a doctor.

"I didn't have a primary care doc in town yet, so I asked around and found one," Daniella recalls. "It took another month to block out an hour when I wasn't in a client meeting, and when I finally saw the doctor, he just agreed that it was allergies and recommended I take my allergy meds more regularly."

Daniella heeded the doctor's advice, but as the summer months passed, her symptoms worsened. Her coughing eventually got so bad she couldn't sleep.

"By that fall I developed a fever, and started feeling short of breath when climbing stairs," Daniella explains. "I was thirty-seven and in great shape, so this made no sense."

When Daniella's symptoms also started including headaches, she figured they were stress related—as she was trying hard to impress her bosses by taking on more cases.

"The headaches were getting more painful, and frequent, but I was way too busy to go see the doctor again," says Daniella. "I just tried to eat healthy, drink lots of water, and plow through it."

Then, one night just before Thanksgiving, Daniella began shaking uncontrollably with what would later be determined was a seizure. When she told the ER doctors she had no history of seizures, they immediately scheduled scans. These revealed a tumor on her brain, and she was admitted to the hospital for a series of tests. Even after studying a brain-tissue sample, doctors could not confirm the exact type of tumor.

"They told me they *thought* it was cancer but were not sure how to proceed," says Daniella. "I had already missed Thanksgiving with my family, when I was going to introduce them to my boyfriend. Now I felt like I was about to lose him, my job, everything. I was terrified."

Daniella called her parents to tell them she "might" have cancer, and they flew in right away to be with her. They insisted their daughter be transferred to a major academic hospital where oncology experts could better assess the situation, and once she was moved, the diagnosis came quickly: Daniella's tumor was the result of lung cancer that had metastasized to her brain. Neither she nor her parents were smokers, and she had never knowingly been exposed to secondhand smoke, asbestos, or other carcinogens, but she had now joined the growing list of early onset lung cancer patients—a group often misdiagnosed by doctors because of their age.

"I couldn't believe this was happening to me," Daniella reflects. "The only people I knew with cancer were my grandparents' age. Now I figured I was probably never even going to get married or have kids, let alone grandkids. And what about my career? Forget about making partner. How could I have the energy to keep working at all?"

Young Adults with Cancer: The Forgotten Group

The "young adult" classification (which is often shortened to "YA" in medical textbooks and journals) can be a confusing one. The guidelines vary among different organizations and institutions, with most categorizing young adults as those aged either fifteen to thirty-nine or eighteen to thirty-nine. For the purposes of this book, we are defining young adult cancer patients as those ages eighteen to forty-nine. Our logic is twofold. Since fifteen- to seventeen-year-olds typically still live at home with their parents, and are not yet legally "adults," they are still being followed by their pediatricians and treated in a pediatric oncology setting. Individuals in their forties, on the other hand, are often going through many of the same transitional life stages as people a few years younger, such as settling down or changing careers, finding a partner, raising children, or caring for aging parents.

This period from when you turn eighteen into your forties is one of tremendous growth, filled with excitement and challenges as you explore who you are and what you want to be. Like it was for Daniella, a cancer diagnosis can feel like a threat not only to your health but also to your future—and your autonomy. If you have children, or want to have them, the potential complications only increase.

Because young adults have just recently begun experiencing cancer in greater numbers, the healthcare community has not yet adapted to their unique medical and psychological needs. As a result, you might feel like you don't belong anywhere. This sensation of not fitting in has its roots in how young adult cancer programs have developed over time. Historically, they grew out of the pediatric oncology world, since these programs already approached care from a developmental perspective and had an understanding of the stages and tasks expected at each age through an individual's adolescence and early twenties. Most pediatric oncology clinics define a patient as a young adult starting at age fifteen, and have both professionals who are well versed in the needs of adolescents as well as programs specifically targeting teenagers. Pediatric oncology is also accustomed to providing family-centered care, and will include services and support for parents, siblings, and extended family and friends.

Adult oncology still had a tendency to lump all adults ages eighteen and older together until 2006, when research studies by the National Cancer Institute (NCI) confirmed that young adults seemed to respond differently to cancer treatment—and at times not as well—when compared to children or older adults with the same cancers.

This data resulted first in a recognition that young adults represent an underserved and vulnerable population, and then a push to include more of them in clinical research.

In the twenty years since then, there has been a continued shift toward an acknowledgment that young adulthood constitutes a different and discrete life stage with unique psychosocial challenges. There is also now an emphasis on long-term follow-up of young adult patients; since individuals in this age group are living longer into survivorship, it is hoped that by studying them, the medical community can better understand the lasting effects of undergoing cancer treatment earlier in life. The media has also played a significant role in bringing attention to this group by highlighting the stories of young adult celebrities with cancer, including some in their late thirties and early forties who have children.

A Growing—and Alarming—Trend

How common is cancer in young adults? According to 2024 American Cancer Society (ACS) statistics, about 80,000 young adults ages twenty to thirty-nine are diagnosed with cancer each year in the United States—accounting for about 4 percent of all cancers diagnosed annually. About 9,000 young adults die from cancer each year, making it the fifth-leading cause of death in this age group, behind accidents, suicide, homicide, and heart disease. It's also the leading cause of death from disease among females ages twenty to thirty-nine, and, for males, is second to heart disease.

Why the Rise in Cases?

Oncologists and cancer researchers are unsure of the reason for this increase in early onset cancers, but the numbers are concerning. As of 2024, for instance, colorectal cancer is the leading cause of cancer deaths for men under fifty—and the second-most common for women in this age group. Breast cancer is the most common cancer in women eighteen to thirty-nine. There are a lot of questions as to why the trend is occurring. A multitude of variables is perhaps contributing to this development:

- It may be genetic differences or mutations that have or have not yet been identified.
- Lifestyle variables including exercise and diet are another possibility, as the rise in early onset cancers has been concurrent with an increase in obesity among young adults—especially in the United States.
- Environmental factors such as pollutants and toxins are likely contributing factors.
- And, perhaps most concerning, is something supported by the experiences of patients like Daniella: Cancers are often not being diagnosed in young adults as early as possible, so the prognosis may not be as good.

Part of the challenge is that young adults do not fit into the typical screening guidelines for cancers not normally associated with their age group. Mammograms to screen for breast cancer are not usually recommended until age forty, and colonoscopies not until forty-five. Such screenings are what help physicians make a diagnosis—most often in the early stages of cancer. While a better understanding of genetic variables and family history has in recent years led the ACS and many other organizations to suggest lowering the recommended screening age, the problem remains that young adults are still being diagnosed with cancers that they and their healthcare providers do not expect.

Cancers previously associated with children, such as neuroblastomas (cancers typically originating in the adrenal glands), are being diagnosed in adults in their twenties and thirties. Because these cancers are so unexpected, it is hard for oncologists and other providers to intervene or to come up with new or revised guidelines. A tremendous amount of basic and clinical research today is focused on trying to categorize and group together the different variables, such as genetics, family history, and lifestyle and environmental factors, in order to devise new guidelines that could lead to earlier diagnoses in young adults.

Another issue is that while the number of young adults with cancer is increasing, the *total* number of these individuals is still low enough to limit our understanding. As stated earlier, just 4 percent of all cancers are diagnosed in people ages twenty to thirty-nine. Even if you look at the oldest group of young adults from the 2022 ACS report statistics—those thirty-five to forty-four—the number rises to just 4.8 percent. For many of the primary care physicians and other health-care providers whose patients fall into these age groups, the percentage of individuals with cancer is small; the thought of such a diagnosis remains under the radar, and is often ruled out.

Understanding the Differences in Treatment Outcome

Despite the alarming trends in young adult incidence, there is some encouraging news about cancer in general: Tremendous advances have been made in cancer treatment during the past half century. According to the ACS, the number of long-term survivors—those living five years or more after diagnosis—has increased from 3 million in 1971 to 12 million in 2012 and more than 18.1 million as of 2024.

The management of side effects caused by treatments has also improved. While nausea during chemotherapy was once so common that patients were routinely handed vomit buckets before their infusions, today there are medications to take beforehand that largely prevent this. Hair loss is also no longer a given, and some treatments actually result in weight *gain* rather than loss. Pain is now addressed beginning at diagnosis and throughout the treatment trajectory, with special medical teams focused on cancer-related pain. Quality of life is also a major consideration today, with nutritional consults, psychosocial care, and integrative therapies such as acupuncture, massage, and meditation that help many patients feel better.

Challenges remain, however. There are different thoughts as to why (as the NCI confirmed in its 2006 findings) young adults respond differently—and often worse—to cancer treatment. Some basic researchers studying colorectal cancer, for instance, believe that there may be something different in the biological makeup of such a cancer when it's diagnosed in younger versus older adults.

But for this and other cancers on the rise in the early onset group, such investigations remain a work in progress. The medical establishment simply does not yet have a full grasp of why—and how—this phenomenon is occurring, or what screening guidelines and lifestyle changes may best work to curtail it.

Factors That Lead to a Late or Missed Diagnosis

Everyone agrees that it would be best if healthcare professionals could determine potential cancer diagnoses as quickly as possible for young adults in their care. Unfortunately, the opposite often occurs. Following are some of the most common reasons for a delayed early onset diagnosis.

Lack of a Long-Standing Relationship with a Doctor

Because many doctors, nurses, and other clinicians see very few, if any, cases of cancer in their eighteen- to forty-nine-year-old patients, they have a tendency to not look for it—even in situations when a simple blood test could either confirm a diagnosis or at least send up a red flag requiring further analysis. As a result, early onset cancers are often misdiagnosed or not caught until they have advanced into a much more serious situation.

It's not *all* the fault of the doctors, though. Part of the issue is steeped in the very nature of young adulthood as a period when individuals are moving away from their families of origin and developing their own lives—and may relocate numerous times due to jobs, college, and other circumstances. They are so busy that many of them don't prioritize annual doctor visits, and they often lack a dedicated primary care physician (PCP) once they "outgrow" their pediatrician.

Contrast this with children under age eighteen, who are still typically under the care of their parents. Most have regular checkups at their pediatricians' offices, and they and their parents tend to develop strong relationships with these doctors over time. Each school year, families are required to submit paperwork ensuring that all their children's vaccines are up-to-date, and some states have additional requirements for students wishing to play sports. Such accountability means that children are routinely seeing their doctors once or twice a year for checkups and blood work, from grade school through high school. In addition, every high fever and broken bone will result in a trip to the pediatrician. Accordingly, there is a far greater likelihood that any major illnesses—including cancer—will be caught early.

Almost immediately after leaving high school, however, newly minted young adults go from having a group of dedicated healthcare advocates to a college or job where *nobody* is looking out for them medically other than their parents noticing a cough or raspy voice during phone calls. I am sure you can relate to this scenario: You start feeling sick or exhausted, and rather than go to bed, or to the doctor, you just attribute it to working too hard, studying too much, or having too much late-night fun with your friends. Some of you in college may not even know where the student health center is located on campus. If you're at a new job in your twenties, you likely only go for annual physicals if your parents remind you.

If you're in your thirties and forties, you are probably more focused on your career, taking *your* children to *their* pediatrician, or caring for elderly parents or grandparents than making your own doctor's appointments. With so many competing demands, your own health is often put on the back burner.

Patient Voices

"As a young woman of color, it took far too long to be diagnosed. My cancer was rare, but it's also because I wasn't truly heard. I almost missed out on more life, more love, and more time with the people who make me feel whole. Cancer already isolates you, but the lack of cultural understanding in healthcare

has a cost. Still, I chose to speak, to create, to keep going. Your
life, your voice, and your purpose still matter." —Shirley J.

Financial Concerns

Finances are another factor in delayed diagnosis. Although many young adults remain covered by their parents' insurance up to the legal age limit of twenty-six, hefty co-pays and the need to submit claims for reimbursement are often enough to turn many of them off from doctor's visits—even for yearly checkups.

Once you're on your own, unless you have a job that provides insurance, you may take a risk and try to do without it. And even if you *do* have insurance, the need to reach high deductibles and cover co-pays may result in proper attention to healthcare losing out to more pressing monetary needs—like car and school payments, rent, and utility bills. Unless you have a partner who effectively takes the place of a nagging parent, things like sudden weight gain or loss or an unexplained spot on your cheek or arm may go unnoticed until they are found to be something worse.

Managing a Young Family

If you are a young adult with kids, you are likely putting your children's medical concerns ahead of your own, just like your parents did, and giving even less attention to a throbbing headache, a persistent cold, or painful joints—all of which could be early indicators of more serious conditions including cancer. Money and time are tighter than ever for young families, and the logistics involved with finding (and paying for) childcare while you make a primary care visit often wind up resulting in no visit at all.

Factoring in Risky Behavior

An additional reason for late diagnosis in the younger age range is that this is a period of life when good health is routinely taken for granted. From age eighteen to thirty, people often feel like they can eat and drink what they want and stay up late partying on work nights and that nothing can stop them. And while young adults typically have a cognitive understanding of life and death, they lack a real emotional grasp of their own mortality. Dying, with the exceptions of wartime, freak accidents, and slasher films, is something that only happens to old people. The thought of death is not usually prominent in this phase of life.

Part of the reason for such an attitude, and a lack of appreciation for the risks and dangers looming out there for *everyone,* can be explained by the development of the human brain. We know that the part of the brain associated with understanding risk, planning ahead, and comprehending the consequences for our behaviors continues to develop until our mid-twenties—and sometimes even a little later than that.

Given these developmental and environmental factors, young adults at times may engage in what could be considered risky behaviors. They either don't quite get the seriousness of such endeavors, or if they do, they understand that risk intellectually—but not behaviorally or emotionally. Some examples include extreme sports like skydiving, exploration of drug use, excessive drinking and vaping, and unprotected sex. All are much more common in this age range, across all socioeconomic classes, and not even those individuals considered "smart" from an intellectual or academic standpoint are immune. Because the emotional and social parts of their brains are still developing, they may not really get how such behaviors can impact their survival. For those a little older, perhaps in the typical age range for having children, the thought of dying and leaving kids behind does not fit our understanding of how life should work.

All of this explains why a cancer diagnosis is such a shock to young adults. In an instant, you are forced to go from thinking that you can do whatever you want to realizing that serious illness and death are *not* such abstract concepts for someone your age.

Feeling Out of Place in Oncology Spaces

Once their cancer is confirmed, young adults soon face another obstacle: feeling out of place at healthcare facilities unaccustomed to dealing with patients like them.

A child under eighteen who is diagnosed with cancer is typically treated in a pediatric oncology clinic, which often has separate areas for babies and toddlers, elementary- and middle school–aged kids, and teenagers. Clinic staff are trained to work with each different group, and to tailor discussion and activities accordingly. Often there are special outreach programs such as day or weekend trips geared specifically to teens under eighteen, who are recognized as a separate developmental age group within the pediatric population.

Young Adult Patients in Spaces Filled with Older People

Those individuals diagnosed at eighteen and older, however, are most often treated with older adults—particularly if they have one of the cancers like breast, colorectal, pancreatic, or lung cancer usually associated with older populations. Have you ever arrived at an oncology appointment, looked around the waiting area, and felt like everybody else wearing a patient wristband resembled your parents or grandparents? Has it seemed like these people were looking at *you* as if you were a caregiver, child, or grandchild accompanying someone to treatment—not a fellow patient? If so, you're not alone. Many of my patients have had the same experiences, where they felt like their own wristbands were all but invisible.

Patient Voices

"Diagnosed at twelve and now living through my fifth recurrence at thirty-three, I've existed as a patient in both the pediatric and adult settings. I went from being stared at for being the oldest in the waiting room to getting the same looks for being the youngest. This transition also meant losing the whole-person pediatric care and entering the adult world, where I needed to be my own coordinator. People stare, questioning how this healthy-looking young adult could have cancer. But this has been my entire life." —Jeremy P.

Young Adult Patients in Spaces Designed for Children

The experience is reversed if you're receiving care in pediatric clinics. This most often occurs when someone in their late teens or early twenties is diagnosed with a cancer commonly found in children, such as a neuroblastoma or specific brain tumors. If you're in this group, you are likely to be assigned to a pediatric oncologist because these doctors are most familiar with the treatment protocol for such cancers. Other families in the waiting area, however, might assume you are either a young parent or older sibling of a child getting treatment. Those who notice your wristband will routinely—and quickly—look away, unsure how to react upon realizing the individual across from them is in fact a patient.

Even the atmosphere and vibe of the typical pediatric clinic feels all wrong for young adults. It is overly bright, filled with toys, art tables, and staff speaking in the happy, high-pitched tones of grade school teachers. While this is an ideal environment to ease the fears of young children who might not totally understand why they are there, it is not the right fit for someone older who knows full well what lies ahead. My patients tell me that while they don't *blame* the well-intentioned staff for acting this way, they can't help but feel unheard and misunderstood. They also feel responsible, as the oldest ones in the clinic, to set an example for the younger patients by being stoic and not expressing their fear or even discomfort with needles and other procedures. In both these situations, the dilemma is the same: Right from the start, even before meeting their care team, they—*you*—already feel isolated and out of place. The great divide that exists between you and your healthy peers, who are charging ahead with their lives while your own life stands still, has extended into the cancer center.

Who Do You Turn To?

A supportive family and/or partner is always very helpful and comforting after a cancer diagnosis, but it's also a complicated situation. Around the time you turned eighteen, you probably began to become more independent from your family of origin and develop your own sense of self. During very early adulthood, your primary support system typically becomes peers going through similar life experiences—you can encourage each other and commiserate over common problems.

A cancer diagnosis throws a wrench into this environment. Even with the rise in early onset cancers, facing such a challenge before age fifty is still quite uncommon. There are usually few—if any—peers who can understand the vulnerable feelings you are suddenly experiencing. Many of my early onset patients tell me that although they believe that their friends care, and *want* to support them, they don't quite seem to know *how*.

As a result, your family of origin may again become part of your day-to-day life. While in some cases the best option for getting help with the tasks of daily living is having parents, siblings, or other close family members move in with you temporarily, in other situations, it might be *you* moving in with *them*. The latter comes with consequences that go beyond the inconvenience of squeezing into the twin bed of your childhood bedroom. After living independently, returning back to your family's care can feel like a form of developmental regression. Even though you are likely extremely thankful for their help, it can be a difficult transition in the midst of an already tumultuous and scary period.

When your mom or dad asks for what feels like the millionth time if you need anything, you might even find yourself lashing out at them. If that's the case, here is something to remember: Your family/caregivers care deeply for you. They will usually understand your mood changes and irritation. You may still feel guilty and know it's unfair to be pushing your anger and frustration onto them, however, because you recognize this situation is also tough on *them*. It's a very difficult dance.

My patients—and their parents—have often described to me a dynamic that develops in the first weeks after diagnosis. Because they are terrified with what is happening, parents sometimes become overly involved in their adult child's care. In some cases they have to, and in other cases it's because they don't know what else *to* do. Regardless of the circumstances, it is challenging for all involved.

If you have a spouse or life partner, their relationship with your family can change too. Your partner might start to feel out of place, and become unsure of how to navigate your relatives or other caregivers, with whom they suddenly have a much different and more intense relationship. Whereas they might have felt on an even playing field with your parents before, it's possible that they could now feel indebted to them, whether for logistical, financial, or other assistance. It all results in a very complicated dynamic, and the awkward combination of dependence and independence can become a source of stress for all involved.

Though there are likely to be some bumps along the way in your relationships post-diagnosis, try not to judge your—and others'—behavior too harshly. Everyone is doing their best in a very difficult situation. We'll talk more about relationships throughout this book, because they are central to all phases of your cancer experience. We will also offer some tips, such as communicating directly and also kindly, that can help smooth out challenging habits or moments.

Looking Ahead

It's clear that a new focus and emphasis on early onset cancer is needed as the number of diagnoses within this age group increases. Your young adult years are a distinct developmental stage of life filled with milestones and challenges that deserve targeted support. Additional medical research, further psychosocial studies, and new patient outreach programs can ensure that patients, their families, oncologists, and other clinicians can continue learning all we can.

In the meantime, you need to focus on your own well-being. Being diagnosed with cancer as a young adult, from eighteen years old through forty-nine, is an unexpected, emotionally traumatic, and consequential life event. This is traditionally a period of dramatic growth—a time to experiment, pursue professional and personal passions, and build your identity as an individual. A cancer diagnosis brings a sudden and shocking halt to the excitement, and you are often left wondering if you will ever be able to regain your momentum—much less handle the myriad financial, logistical, and other challenges to come. These are very common fears, and I hope the rest of this book can reassure you that you're not alone while offering suggestions on how to best manage your journey.

Key Points

- The number of young people in the US with cancer is rising. We don't know for sure the reasons for the trend, but it could be related to genetic, lifestyle, environmental, and other factors.
- Early onset cancer diagnoses are often missed or delayed, perhaps because of skipped annual physicals, symptoms being ignored, or barriers like lack of health insurance.
- Spaces like oncologist offices and waiting rooms—and many cancer-treatment programs themselves—are usually tailored either to children or to older adults, leaving young adults feeling out of place.
- A cancer diagnosis changes your relationships with those around you, even well-meaning parents, friends, and loved ones.

CHAPTER 2

Early Days

At first, Greg figured he was just working too hard. He was, after all, a twenty-two-year-old college student racing to finish his senior thesis while also juggling five classes and a part-time job. So when he started feeling very tired, having night sweats, and developing itchy skin, he chalked it up to his demanding lifestyle and how he was coping with it.

"I had been drinking more than usual as a way of relaxing and trying to have some fun," Greg recalls. "Since the symptoms seemed exacerbated by alcohol, I thought maybe my body was reacting badly to all the drinking. I stopped, but it didn't help."

Eventually, after nagging from his girlfriend, Greg went to the campus health center. A nurse there said his problems were likely caused by stress, and suggested that he take a few days to rest and ask professors for extensions on his work. A few days later, when Greg noticed swelling in his neck, he decided to go to an off-campus urgent care center—where a doctor said his lymph nodes were likely enlarged due to an infection and gave him antibiotics.

"The antibiotics didn't help, and it got to where I was so sick I couldn't even function," explains Greg. "When I went home for spring break, my mom made me go see my old pediatrician."

The pediatrician ordered a complete workup, and Greg spent several days getting various tests done. Then he was called to come back in—this time with his parents. Greg was curious but not overly concerned. Maybe his childhood doctor was planning to lecture him in front of his folks about not burning the candle at both ends.

Then he heard: The initial workup suggested it may be cancer.

Upon the mention of that word—"cancer"—Greg became so frightened that he couldn't even hear what the doctor said next about seeing an oncologist and likely needing chemotherapy. His heart was racing, he had difficulty breathing, his hands were shaking, and he became overwhelmed with emotion.

"I couldn't remember the last time I had cried, but these feelings were like nothing I'd experienced before, and I just couldn't stop them," says Greg. "I'm thankful my parents were there asking questions and taking notes for me, because I felt out of control and helpless. At the same time, I also felt weirdly relieved—at least I finally had an answer for why I had been feeling so sick."

Within the next several weeks, Greg was diagnosed with Hodgkin lymphoma (cancer of the lymph system). During this time, he regularly found his mind wandering. The constant texts and phone calls from family and friends only added to the stress. He understood they cared and meant well, but it was just too much. Once Greg's frustration led him to start snapping at people, he chose to avoid them altogether and bury himself in schoolwork and his job.

"If I didn't keep busy, I would start picturing myself bald and worrying about how others would perceive me," Greg explains.

Even though Greg's oncologist assured him that Hodgkin lymphoma was a "curable" cancer and that he would resume his busy life in time, it didn't quell his fears and anxiety.

"I was already unlucky enough to get cancer in the first place, something that shouldn't happen to a person my age," Greg remembers thinking. "What if the treatment didn't work for me?"

Riding the Emotional Roller Coaster

Being diagnosed with cancer is a tremendously emotional experience. A few of the many emotions you might encounter are shock, denial, disbelief, terror, anxiety, worry, sadness, anger, helplessness, hopelessness, and confusion.

Patients often ask, "Is it normal to be scared, angry, and depressed, sometimes all at the same time?" My answer is yes. If you were *not* distraught in such a situation, then I would be worried. It's completely natural to be terrified upon hearing the word "cancer" in connection to your health. Some patients experience emotions they didn't expect—for example, like Greg, you might feel a sense of relief after getting a diagnosis, because it provides an explanation for why you feel so awful.

Also as in Greg's case, it's common to undergo an onslaught of various emotions and fears immediately upon getting such news. The period from when a person learns they have cancer until their first treatment typically takes two to eight weeks, and during this time most young adults report feeling as if they are on an emotional roller coaster. You're often waiting for tests and scans to come back that will determine the extent of your cancer, and living with the uncertainty can be excruciating.

You don't yet know exactly what you are going to be coping with. Is the cancer confined to one part of your body? Has it spread locally, or is it in other organs? Just how advanced is it? As you ponder the possibilities, all of them frightening, you can find yourself overwhelmed with anxiety, worry, and racing thoughts. Patients sometimes say they are in so much fear that they can't even get out of bed as they try to assimilate all this information.

When it comes to interacting with loved ones, newly diagnosed patients can feel wound up, irritable, and angry—often simultaneously. You know your family and friends are there to support you, and are trying to be kind, but you might feel like telling them to leave you alone rather than deal with answering the same questions over and over again. Sometimes it just feels like it's too much effort to process it all, and your patience can suffer as a result.

At times you may also be overcome with sadness, and find yourself crying and thinking about your life. You might wonder, "Am I going to make it through this? Could I die? And if I die, what will that do to my family?" Then, at other times, the sadness might turn to anger and frustration. Here the question becomes: "Why is this happening to me—and why at this point in my life? Why do I have to deal with this at my age?" It can be a hard thing to wrap your head around.

Even if you don't count yourself among the many new cancer patients who think, "Why me?"—a completely acceptable question—it can be extremely hard to focus, concentrate, and assimilate information after you're initially diagnosed. You may find yourself struggling to get work done, because you're *consumed* with thinking about your cancer. Everything seems like a great unknown, and feeling sad thoughts and crying are common. Some people lose their appetite, while others can't stop eating. You might feel like crawling into bed and pulling up the covers, but sleep can be elusive—even when you're exhausted.

Patient Voices

"One week after diagnosis, I wrote, It's been a week filled with a lot of emotions; scared, angry, overwhelmed, anxious, but above all, a feeling of being truly blessed. I remember feeling like a deer in headlights, wide-eyed and overwhelmed with every new person I met, every test I had to endure, and every new piece of information I received. But I was also completely flooded with love from family and friends, and in amazement of the compassionate care I was receiving from doctors, nurses, and social workers." —Jessica S.

Then, on top of it all, is the sense of shock and denial. It's hard to believe this is really happening to you. Some patients tell me they have moments when they start reading or watching TV or playing a video game, and they are able to go into a state of hyperfocus or distraction—forgetting momentarily what they are going through. Then, of course, everything comes rushing back.

The key thing to know at this point is that *all of these emotions are understandable*. You know you have cancer, but there are likely still so many unknowns: the extent of the cancer and your prognosis, the details of your upcoming treatment, the possible side effects, and how you are going to deal with it all. While these feelings of anxiety and fear can be extremely uncomfortable, they can also be useful—and have been of service to humans since long before anybody knew about cancer.

Understanding Your Stone Age Brain

In terms of evolution, humans have been equipped to face threats to our well-being and lives since our cave-dwelling days. These automatic, adaptive responses were then used to help us survive dangerous situations—such as an animal attacking. The body readied itself to fight the threat, to flee or run from it, or to freeze (when facing predators such as snakes or big cats that respond to movement).

The same responses present themselves today, whether you are facing an oncoming car at a crosswalk or receiving a cancer diagnosis. Physiologically, your body prepares to defend you against the threat to your life. I like to refer to the process as tapping into your Stone Age brain. Think of that car, or that cancer, as a saber-toothed tiger bearing down on you. Your body's automatic response to save you means all your energy is redirected to help you fight or flee from the threat.

Here are some of the common reactions I've heard described by patients facing a new cancer diagnosis, along with why it is adaptive to the fight-or-flight response:

- **Racing heart:** The heart is pumping faster to more quickly get blood and oxygen to major muscles (leg, thigh, arm muscles) necessary to fight or flee (or sometimes flee and then hide/freeze).
- **Breathing changes/shortness of breath:** The big muscles in our bodies (usually in our legs, thighs, and arms) need more oxygen and blood flow to help us confront or run from danger, and these changes ensure we get it.
- **Muscle tightness:** Our big muscles tighten as more blood flows to them and prepares us to pounce into action. This can result in aches and pains, especially if we don't run or flee.
- **Tingling fingers:** Since our fingers are usually not needed when confronting a major threat, there is less blood flow to them—resulting in a tingling, numbing sensation.
- **Gastrointestinal distress:** The body does not need to focus on digestion when confronting a potentially life-threatening

situation, so resources are redirected away from that system. As a result, you may experience dry mouth, nausea, vomiting, or literally be "scared shitless" with diarrhea.

- **Urinary urgency:** Again, under extreme stress, the muscles in your bladder relax. This explains why some people urinate on themselves when facing a threat to their lives.
- **Sweating and clamminess:** It takes a lot of effort and resources to prepare for a threat, and sweating is a way for the body to cool off. It also makes you slippery if someone tries to grab you!
- **Lightheadedness:** The key at this time is to not overthink or be indecisive. Action is imperative, so oxygen is being forced to our big muscles. That means there is slightly less of it available for our brains. This is not a dangerously low amount of oxygen; just a way of redirecting the body's resources to where they are most needed.

These explanations offer an understanding of why you may have some or all of these reactions upon your diagnosis: You are receiving information that presents a potential threat to your life. I hope they can provide reassurance that your body is doing what it should to protect you.

Many of my patients experience a whole new wave of panic when they notice these physical reactions. They think, "Am I having a heart attack now, in addition to having cancer?" No, they are not. While you can't literally physically fight or flee your cancer like you would a saber-toothed tiger or onrushing car, your body still responds this way. Humans have not yet evolved to react differently to threats in the environment that they can run from or physically overpower versus those that, while just as real and immediate—such as a serious illness, *can't* be dealt with that way.

When you're feeling particularly vulnerable, try to remember that what you're experiencing is normal for someone facing a frightening and threatening situation—and while it may feel uncomfortable, you *will* get through it. In later chapters, we will discuss ways to help manage these feelings of anxiety and fear.

Beware Dr. Google

While you may be tempted to go blindly seeking answers online about your diagnosis in an attempt to quell fears and uncertainty about what lies ahead, do your best to avoid going down this rabbit hole. Only your oncology team truly understands *your* cancer. I have so many young adults come to sessions overwhelmed with anxiety about something they find online. More often than not, the information is either from an unreliable source, outdated, too general (and therefore nonapplicable to their specific cancer)—or a combination of all three.

Even if research found online is reported as having been published "this year," it is likely *not* the most current findings. Most published research is the result of investigators tracking patients for a number of years to provide accurate response-to-treatment or survival data. By the time those findings have been published, there are already *new* studies being conducted with new agents and new clinical trials.

As you may have learned upon receiving what initially seemed like a specific type of cancer diagnosis—such as leukemia or sarcoma—even these cancers are subdivided. There are, for example, several different *types* of leukemia, such as acute lymphocytic leukemia (ALL), acute myeloid leukemia (AML), and chronic lymphocytic leukemia (CLL), as well as various different sarcomas. There is not just one type of lymphoma or brain tumor either, so it is important to keep in mind that treatments are tailored to the very distinct type of cancer you have. The NCI and ACS have very robust websites, but they may not have the detailed information needed to learn all you want about your specific cancer as it relates to young adults. Again—your oncology team knows your diagnosis and individual situation best. Writing down questions for your team and bringing these to your appointments is the best way to get accurate information.

One note of caution I feel is important to mention here: While it's great that there is a growing number of young adults sharing their cancer journeys online through social media posts, personal blogs, and YouTube testimonials, be wary about taking advice they might provide. Everybody has their own ideas about what works best for them, but you should never try *any* approach—medical, nutritional, holistic, or otherwise—without first running it by your oncologist. If you think some of the tips or insights from fellow cancer patients sound promising, write them down to share with your team.

Second Opinions

If you have gotten a diagnosis from a well-regarded or recommended medical facility, you might wonder whether it is necessary to get a second opinion somewhere else. In short: Yes, it's usually a good idea.

As we have discussed, young adult cancers are not common—and going for a second opinion at one of the many NCI-Designated Cancer Centers can be critical to your care. In addition, if you have been diagnosed with a rare or uncommon type of cancer, it's especially important to try to get a second opinion at such a facility with oncologists experienced in treating rare cancers. These centers all receive NCI funding to deliver the most up-to-date cancer treatments to patients based on their laboratory and clinical research. Research suggests that being seen at an NCI-Designated Cancer Center, especially one focused on young adults with cancer, can actually impact chances of long-term survival for patients in this age group. Don't worry about letting one potential oncologist know you're seeking a second opinion; this is a sensible and entirely reasonable thing to do.

Even if you do not live close enough to an NCI center to receive all your treatment there, consider getting a second opinion. Some NCI facilities, although not all, offer the option of virtual visits for second opinions, and will review records and test results sent over by another clinical team. A distant oncology team can guide your care closer to home, and also keep you informed about new treatments, their availability, and access to clinical trials—research studies in which human subjects are given new drugs or drug combinations to test their safety and effectiveness against established treatments.

Learning a New Language

Before your treatment actually starts, the biggest challenge is often not becoming totally overwhelmed. There is so much going on—and so much information being thrown at you—that it may be hard to process everything.

Patients often tell me that when they first start going over their treatment plans, and hearing the names of which specific chemotherapy, immunotherapy, or radiation course they might be getting, it all becomes very confusing. Many don't know the difference between one treatment and another, and it can feel like trying to learn a whole new language. In reality, that's what it is. Even my patients who are physicians themselves are unsure of what's what if they don't specialize in oncology. The names of the drugs are unfamiliar, and there are so many new treatments constantly coming out that it is impossible for anybody not providing that specialized care to know them. One suggestion I give to all my patients is that they keep notes—on paper or on their phones—of any new terms, treatments, or drugs they learn about, and go over these with their team. You should do this too; think of it as your "cancer dictionary."

Finding a Doctor Who's a Good Match for You

Another strategy that can help you feel more confident as you navigate the early days of your diagnosis is to become an educated medical consumer. If you're going to buy a car, or a house, you get information; you ask experts; you try out or get a feel for what you're buying. If you're looking for a new restaurant, or visiting a new city, you read reviews and look at photos before deciding where to go. But when it comes to unique medical care, there is no Yelp or Fodor's guide to help.

This task is also one part of the cancer journey that is particularly challenging for young adults. Many healthcare professionals working in the cancer setting have limited, if any, experience dealing with this age group. The problem has only increased in recent years as breast, colorectal, and lung cancers have become more common among those ages eighteen to forty-nine. Now clinicians must deal not only with young adults facing cancers typically associated with both their age group and children, like sarcomas and leukemias, but also those diagnosed with what have traditionally been considered cancers of middle-aged and older adults.

It's important to keep in mind as you seek out the best oncology center and care team that most cancers have very specific protocols and treatment plans shown to be effective for that cancer. The National Comprehensive Cancer Network (NCCN), a not-for-profit alliance of leading US cancer centers focused on patient care, research, and education, has also established explicit treatment guidelines. There are NCCN guidelines and protocols to follow for all types of cancers, and these are carried out at healthcare facilities nationwide.

That said, it's vital to make sure your potential oncologist is familiar with not just cancer, but *your type* of cancer. There is a lot of variability, even within NCI-Designated Cancer Centers, but by posing some questions—to yourself and the specialist—you can find out if a doctor is a good match.

Questions to Ask Yourself

One of the biggest keys to finding the right specialist is how you feel when talking with that person. This is something you can usually get a handle on by asking yourself some basic questions about them:

- Do they take time to answer your questions?
- Do they understand and support your concerns?
- Do they look you in the eye when talking to you?
- How do they interact with you? With respect, or do they talk down to you?
- Do they or their team follow up after your appointments to see how you are doing?

All these things are important to think about, because this person is going to be a big part of your life for the foreseeable future.

You need to know you can trust them, respect them, and be yourself around them.

Questions to Ask the Doctor

I suggest asking questions of your clinical team before the start of treatment. In fact, think of it as a job interview. If you're hiring someone, you're looking for the best candidate to work with—someone who understands your company's products or services and knows all about how they function. It's the same with you and your cancer, only in this case, the interviewee's knowledge of the "product" could have potentially life-altering implications.

Another factor in these interactions is that your understandably heightened anxiety can interfere with your ability to remember and assimilate information. To mitigate that challenge, write down your questions and bring along a family member or friend (or have them join virtually) to help you record or recall the information provided.

For example, say you have just received a colorectal cancer diagnosis. You can learn the degree of specialization a doctor has in this specific cancer—or whatever cancer you have—by asking questions like these up front:

- "What is your experience treating colorectal cancer?"
- "Do you *only* treat colorectal cancer, or do you also treat stomach cancer and other types of gastrointestinal (GI) cancers?"
- "How many other types of cancers outside of GI do you treat?"
- "What is your experience treating *young adults* with colorectal cancer?"
- "Do you offer access to clinical trials here?"

Remember that the same cancer can behave differently—and respond differently to treatment—when it appears in the young adult population versus in a pediatric or older adult patient. Maybe an oncologist you are considering has a great deal of experience in colorectal cancer but hasn't treated a lot of young adults with it. That's why this specific question is so important.

Don't feel self-conscious about asking too many questions of the oncologists you meet with. These are all normal inquiries that doctors should *expect* to be asked, especially around something as serious as cancer. If an oncologist becomes in any way defensive in response to your queries, and/or is unable or reluctant to answer them, that's cause for concern as well—and something you want to keep in mind as you proceed with choosing and maintaining your clinical team.

These "interviews" when seeking an oncology team are also good practice in terms of becoming more comfortable advocating for yourself—a skill that will help you throughout your cancer journey. After all, it's *your* life. You need to find the place, and the people, who are going to give you the best possible care and comfort.

Patient Voices

"Finding the right treatment team began with trusting my instinct to seek a life-changing second opinion. That critical second opinion came before my diagnosis, when I insisted on having agonizing fibroids removed rather than continuing to wait. Hidden behind the fibroids, cancer was discovered. I was diagnosed with a rare cancer typically found in children and was referred to a specialist trained in both pediatric and adult cancer. I didn't need to search endlessly for the right doctors; the nature of the cancer led me directly to them." —Deja W.

Sharing Your Personal Preferences

Everybody has their own comfort zone when it comes to doctor's office dynamics. Maybe you're so anxious when you come in for appointments that you hate any initial chitchat—you just want your test results, blood counts, or whatever news you're waiting for before discussing anything else. Or maybe you *like* when your doctor starts appointments by asking how you're doing, what you've been up to, and if you are experiencing any problems or side effects. Since you know they will eventually get around to telling you your results, you're okay with waiting a bit. Some people like lots of details when getting results, and others prefer general information and fewer details.

Whichever way, don't be afraid to share your preferences with your care team. Sometimes a little bit of coaching on your part can be helpful in making these interactions work even better for you. For example, try asking, "Can you do it this way for me instead? It makes me feel better." You'll find most doctors will try to be more accommodating.

Leaning on Other Members of a Care Team

Sometimes you may find an accomplished oncologist who's a specialist in your particular diagnosis, but you don't feel totally comfortable with them for one reason or another. In those cases, see if there is someone else on their treatment team who you connect with better. Maybe that's a nurse practitioner or physician assistant who works closely with the oncologist and could meet with you at your regular appointments. The oncologist would still be overseeing your overall care, but you'd be able to build a strong bond and communication with this other member of the team.

Think of it this way: If you've found an oncologist who has expertise in your cancer, you may not want to lose them. You can benefit from the doctor's proficiency and still feel at ease during your appointments. It's the *team* that you are selecting, not just the oncologist, and all of them want what works best for you. Of course, if you really don't feel comfortable with your oncologist, it is perfectly fine to change to a different doctor within the same center—or even go to another institution entirely. You need to make the best decisions for you.

Thinking Ahead: How and When Cancer Impacts Fertility

Why bring up fertility when you've just been handed a life-changing cancer diagnosis? Because many cancer treatments can be potentially toxic to your reproductive health—and reproduction typically happens in early adulthood. Even if having children is not something on your mind right now, it's important to understand the fertility risks associated with each aspect of treatment: surgery, chemotherapy, targeted therapies, immunotherapy, and radiation. The possibility of infertility is yet another way that cancer is threatening to disrupt your life—but there are things you can do about it.

What Is Oncofertility?

The term "oncofertility" was coined in 2006 by research scientist Teresa Woodruff, PhD, an expert in ovarian biology and reproductive science, to describe a merging of the fields of oncology and fertility. Woodruff's belief, which has since been championed by the NCI and National Institutes of Health (NIH), is that cancer specialists and reproductive specialists should collaborate in a joint mission to help patients and their families understand how cancer can impact fertility—and make decisions accordingly.

As the number of cancer cases among young adults has sharply increased in recent years, this evolving discipline has become more important than ever. Before oncofertility consults became a widely accepted part of cancer care, there was no regular process for connecting patients with fertility specialists. If cancer patients wanted to explore in vitro fertilization, for instance, they often went to the same clinic as the general population—and were put on waiting lists they could not afford to be on. Today, if a cancer patient wishes to explore fertility-preservation options, they are linked up by their oncologist to a reproductive medicine team in the same or a partnering facility. In fact, there are guidelines now put out by the American Society of Clinical Oncology (ASCO), European Society for Medical Oncology, and the American Society for Reproductive Medicine recommending that fertility options be discussed with cancer patients.

The knowledge and situations surrounding oncofertility can vary dramatically from patient to patient. I've seen twenty-one-year-olds who come into treatment having already given thought to their fertility, or in some cases who already have a child. There are other patients of the same age, however, who tell me that they had not yet considered parenthood. Even if a patient is in their late twenties, that can still be the case. After all, they explain, they're still young. They may very much want kids, they may even know *how many* they want, but they are just not ready yet. Others have a child, or multiple children, and think they may want more in the future. Still others may not want children at all.

Sometimes I see cancer survivors on the "older end" of young adulthood, maybe thirty-nine or forty, and they'll express something called "decision regret." They didn't decide about oncofertility when they *could* have, and are now wondering why they didn't contemplate it more. Yes, they were informed that their cancer treatment may in some ways be toxic to their fertility, but at the time they did not pay attention. That's why it's essential that whatever your current circumstances or future planning might be, you try and give thought to oncofertility when possible.

There are new oncofertility options emerging all the time, which is why it's so important to ask your oncology team if the fertility experts they work with are truly knowledgeable about oncofertility and the latest trends in the field. With all this in mind, I believe you should strongly consider seeking out psychological support during this time. If such help is not offered by your oncology team, ask for it. Even before actually starting fertility treatment, you might want to consult with a therapist who is knowledgeable in this area to review your options and get assistance with treatment decision-making. Receiving impartial guidance about what is best for you as an individual can be very valuable. Of course, if you have a partner, depending on the specific circumstances, their input and involvement is critically important as well.

Potential Effects of Common Treatments on Fertility

There are things that can be done today to try and help prevent infertility around different treatments, but it's important to know potential impacts ahead of time. Here is some key information to know:

- **Chemotherapy:** During chemotherapy, multiple factors are at play, including the type of chemotherapy, the dosage, the frequency and length of treatment, and your age. In terms of drugs, the highest risk for infertility in male and female patients occurs with a group of drugs known as alkylating agents—such as cyclophosphamide, ifosfamide, temozolomide, busulfan, chlorambucil, melphalan, and procarbazine. FOLFOX and cisplatin also present risk, but less so. It is not guaranteed that any of these drugs will *cause* infertility, but they do put you at increased risk for it. As always, it's important to discuss with your oncology team beforehand the risks associated with whatever drugs and regimen you are undergoing and make an informed decision.

- **Targeted therapies and immunotherapies:** A new area of cancer treatment to emerge in recent years and receive lots of attention is that of targeted therapies and immunotherapies. These treatments have made a huge difference in helping patients live longer and with good quality of life. We don't know quite as much as we'd like to yet about how they impact fertility, because they are still so new—and more of them are being developed all the time. One such treatment, Avastin, has been shown in a study to negatively impact fertility. But more research certainly needs to be done.

- **Radiation therapy:** The damage radiation can cause to your fertility depends on a host of variables, including the dose of radiation you are receiving, the area that is being radiated, and the type of radiation. Often people are very aware of the potential danger; for instance, if they are receiving radiation to their pelvic area, it makes sense that this might damage their fertility.

  It is not always so obvious or logical, however. Fertility is much more complicated than that. It can also be an issue if the radiation is to your central nervous system, and hormones that are secreted by different parts of our bodies are critically important to our fertility. Treatment for gastrointestinal cancers like colorectal cancer, and, of course, total body radiation—which may be used when undergoing a bone marrow transplant—also carry a risk. So no matter what type of radiation you are receiving, remember to always ask questions.

- **Surgery:** As with radiation, if surgery is being done to an organ associated with reproduction—like an ovary, cervix, or uterus—doctors (and patients) tend to understand the potential impact on fertility. Still, it is important to ask questions like, "If you are taking a cancerous ovary out, will you be leaving the other one in?" or "Based on the type of surgery I am having, is there a way you can be conservative with the procedure, still get the best treatment outcome, but also preserve my fertility and reproductive ability?"

    For testicular cancer, fertility is in most cases not a factor, because the patient usually still has one testis left. There are times, however, when a patient with *metastatic* testicular cancer needs to have chemotherapy in addition to surgery. In these instances it's important to bring up fertility, because men can bank their sperm before chemotherapy and hopefully have children later on if they want. If you have a prostate cancer diagnosis, you should also ask your doctor how treatment will impact your fertility.

    At times an organ that you would never think of being involved with fertility can actually influence reproduction. In the case of colorectal cancer, for instance, there are certain situations when the type of surgery that *needs* to be done—the surgery that gives you the best chance at survival—can also have an impact on your fertility. Again, it's best to ask.

Barriers to Oncofertility

There are at least four major barriers standing in the way of a patient accessing oncofertility options:

1. **Patient knowledge:** This is a good argument for why it's so important to use reliable sources affiliated with an agency like the NCI or NIH when seeking information about your cancer. A lot of patients are simply not aware until it's too late

of the toxic nature of cancer treatment and how it can impact their ability to have children.

2. **Clinician communication skills:** Especially if they have not previously treated many young adult patients, oncologists and their teams can struggle with how to ask early onset patients about fertility. In some extreme cases, clinicians themselves may not know the exact potential toxicity of the treatment they are readying to provide, even though there are very strict guidelines urging oncologists to let their patients know this is part of their overall care. Even well-versed clinicians aware of the serious impact cancer treatment can have on an individual's fertility may struggle to communicate these risks with a patient effectively.

3. **Connecting with specialists:** Unfortunately, not all cancer-treatment facilities have access to and/or working relationships with reproductive health specialists, much less ones who specialize in oncofertility. This is why it's so important for patients to be connected with experts who are best equipped to help them understand different oncofertility options—and share new alternatives as they become available.

4. **Cost:** The cost for fertility treatments and preservation (storage) can be substantial, especially for female patients, although assistance is often available. Costs can vary quite a bit depending on the facility being used, your insurance provider and plan, and the part of the country in which you are accessing them. Some patients may have fewer resources to draw from and less access to insurance that might cover some of the costs. In the Resources section of this book, we have listed organizations and foundations that can be of assistance with fertility-preservation costs. In addition, many of the academic medical centers have specialists and staff who routinely deal with young adult patients and can provide a great deal of guidance in getting you to those resources.

Working with both an oncologist and a reproductive health specialist right from the start is essential when considering oncofertility options, because going this route will likely require a delay in the start of your cancer treatment. The fears associated with deferring treatment can be real, so you should consult with both your oncologist and a reproductive specialist to see if your circumstances allow for fertility preservation prior to treatment. New methods for fertility preservation are being researched and approved on a continuous basis, so it is important that *all* options and related concerns are presented and talked about in an honest, open manner. If your treatment needs to start immediately as a result of a particular diagnosis, that should be part of the discussion. There may still be an oncofertility option open to you, and your oncologist should be willing to offer it.

Historically Marginalized Populations

Patients who are not heterosexual, white, and cisgender might experience additional hurdles. For example, if you are a member of the LGBTQ+ community, you need to be extra aware of the possibility that oncofertility options may not be presented appropriately to you. Even in an era of more inclusive cancer care, in which the number of openly gay, lesbian, bisexual, and transgender oncology patients is higher than ever, a subtle form of discrimination known as unconscious bias—snap judgments we make about people and situations based on subconscious socialization and stereotyping—still occurs. Well-meaning oncologists may withhold information without even realizing it, so it's essential that you be ready for this possibility and speak up if you feel you are not being given appropriate oncofertility guidance.

Members of certain ethnic, racial, and religious groups should also be on the lookout for unconscious bias. Patients in religious groups known for having strong feelings about the preservation of embryos have also been on the receiving end of subtle discrimination from clinicians who assume such patients would never consider fertility preservation.

No matter how a clinician may feel personally, such behavior is wrong. Whether or not they are aware they are doing it, withholding *any* type of information from patients based on preconceived notions can have a detrimental impact on their care. Open, unbiased discussion is the key to avoiding such situations. As unfair as it may seem, patients need to advocate for themselves by speaking up and asking questions.

In the end, what's important is not just whether a certain means of fertility preservation is available, and what steps are involved with that process, but also that you feel you have different options to consider. It's your life, and your body, so you need all the information and understanding you can gather to make the best choice for you. That's why strong communication and collaboration between you, your oncologist, and the reproductive specialist is essential. As with all aspects of cancer treatment, you are your own best advocate.

What's Involved with Male Fertility Preservation

The main way for men to engage in fertility preservation is through sperm collection and banking. This is something that can be done easily and quickly, usually within a couple of days. Once your oncology team sets up your appointment, you just go in and provide a sperm sample through ejaculation, and it gets banked (or frozen) for future use. If time allows, you might want to collect samples on two or three separate days. The sperm bank will store the sperm until you are ready to have a child.

What's Involved with Female Fertility Preservation

While a male patient usually only needs to delay cancer treatment for a few days, a female patient needs to wait until their eggs are retrieved—a process that requires additional treatment to make those eggs mature and become available for retrieval.

Once your eggs have matured, an outpatient surgical procedure is needed to retrieve them and ready the eggs for the next step. Depending on your individual situation, this can sometimes be difficult. Knowing your options, and what can be done, is critical in these cases. Sometimes, if a fertility specialist is used to working with female cancer patients, they may have protocols in place that can speed up the process so a patient can begin treatment sooner. Then, after your eggs have been retrieved, you have two main choices of what to do:

1. The eggs can be frozen through cryopreservation and then, like sperm, preserved until needed.
2. You can undergo in vitro fertilization (IVF), in which sperm is used to fertilize your eggs and form embryos, which are then frozen. You could use a partner's or donor's sperm to form the embryos.

In cases where you are receiving radiation to your pelvic area, the ovaries can often be moved outside the radiation field in a surgical process called ovarian transposition. Sometimes surgeons can even move ovarian tissue and still preserve a patient's fertility, so it's important to explore these options up front with your radiation oncology team.

Often, females with leukemia or other cancers for which treatment must start immediately may be placed on a medicine that stops menstruation, such as Lupron, *during* their cancer treatment. There is some thought that by stopping menstruation, and preserving some of those eggs from being released, it could preserve fertility once treatment is over. Research is so far inconclusive; although menstruation does usually restart after their treatment is over and they stop taking Lupron, that does not necessarily mean their fertility will always be preserved.

Be Gentle with Yourself

Being diagnosed with cancer as a young adult is an unexpected and extremely frightening experience. Remember, this is a period filled with major developmental milestones, when you are building a sense of identity, gaining independence, and growing academically, professionally, and in your peer and intimate relationships. Cancer interrupts—and disrupts—all of it.

As you deal with the range of emotional and physical responses your body undergoes after diagnosis, be gentle with yourself. Try not to judge your reactions; simply notice and accept what you are experiencing. Your journey with cancer will take time, and you may feel especially vulnerable and overwrought in these early days.

Greg, the college student we heard from in the chapter opening, struggled with processing information and trying to make decisions after his diagnosis. Understandably overwhelmed, he found it difficult to answer questions from family and friends. In the next chapter, we will start by examining how to communicate information to your loved ones in ways that are manageable for you and sensitive to all concerned.

Key Points

- In the first moments, and days, after learning they have cancer, most young adults undergo a roller coaster of emotions and physical sensations. Sometimes several can happen simultaneously, or they can alternate back and forth. You may often feel out of control, which—given the situation—is totally understandable.
- Avoid googling information after your diagnosis. It is unlikely that what you find will pertain to people in your age group who have your particular cancer, nor will it be up-to-date. It's best to go to the experts—your oncology team—with questions and concerns; don't rely on Dr. Google.
- Finding the best oncology team to treat your specific cancer is important, and may require traveling for treatment or to get a second opinion (often a good idea). Anxiety can interfere with your ability to remember specific details, so when possible, have a family member or friend accompany you to your oncology visits to help you recall things.
- While advocating for yourself as a young adult may not be easy, initially asking questions and addressing specific concerns—such as the impact of cancer treatment on your fertility—is important.

CHAPTER 3

Sharing the News and Next Steps

Maria first felt the lump on her left breast one morning while showering. The hair salon where she worked did not provide health insurance, so when the bump didn't go away after a few weeks, she got it checked at a community clinic. Because she was just thirty-one, and had no family history of breast cancer, Maria was told the lump was likely due to hormonal changes.

"My friend who was a nurse convinced me to go to a diagnostic breast center," explains Maria. "They had me undergo a mammogram, ultrasound, and biopsy, and diagnosed me with breast cancer."

The center referred Maria to a surgeon, but she was too scared to go. She felt paralyzed and confused by the situation. Being so young, and without any cancer history in her family, she didn't understand how this could be happening. One of Maria's older customers was a breast cancer survivor, so she confided in her. The customer suggested Maria go to a university-affiliated cancer center, where they had terrific doctors and treated patients of all ages. It was a forty-five-minute drive, but Maria wanted to get the best care possible. Her mother and sister went to the appointment with her to provide emotional support.

The breast cancer team there explained that because the cancer was still small, Maria had two surgical options: a lumpectomy or a mastectomy. If she got the lumpectomy, she would require radiation afterward; if she got the mastectomy, she got to decide if she wanted immediate reconstruction (and if so, what type). Either way, she would likely need chemotherapy after surgery.

"It was hard to keep track of all the different doctors and everything they were telling us," recalls Maria. "It was a lot to take in."

Things got even more overwhelming when Maria's large extended family, friends, and salon customers learned of her diagnosis and started calling, texting, and emailing. Many said they were praying for her, and a few even had suggestions on supplements or herbs to "wipe out the cancer." Maria was grateful for the messages, but just the thought of replying to each one made her tired.

Thankfully, a social worker at the cancer center suggested Maria assign someone in her family, perhaps her sister (who came to all her appointments), to send out group texts with updates. This made Maria feel a lot better, and comfortable opening up to the social worker about another concern.

"I told her I sometimes used to vape with my friends, and was worried that had caused the cancer," says Maria. "She urged me to share this with my medical team, and said that nobody would judge me for it. She also reassured me that occasional vaping was not likely to be associated with breast cancer."

When Maria next mentioned the supplements and herbs people had recommended, the social worker suggested she check them out with the center's integrative medicine department. Maria did, and wound up not using any of them. She went ahead with a lumpectomy, radiation, and chemotherapy.

Spreading the Word to Other Adults

Up to this point, you have probably been going through tests and waiting, both for a diagnosis and to know more about what will happen next. During this time, of course, many of the people who love and care about you, as well as others with whom you have daily contact—like coworkers—may also be wondering what's going on.

One thing I commonly hear from patients is that they feel nervous and on edge in the early stages of treatment. Like Maria, they are trying to process all this information, understand it, and then make decisions.

It's hard in such a situation to have the wherewithal, energy, and cognitive focus needed to talk with others about your cancer. The exception are those closest to you, who you've likely already told. They may even have been going with you to your first appointments and helping keep track of all the key details shared by your clinical team. *They* know the story, and what's coming next, but everyone else is still in the dark.

Major events like a cancer diagnosis bring to light just how many different people most of us are connected to in the various areas of our lives. These contacts may be social- or work- or school-related, or even the parents of our children's friends. It's hard and time-consuming to communicate individually with each and every one of them, and exhausting to have to repeat the information over and over. On top of that, as you're telling the story of your diagnosis, you're often *reliving it*, which can be very mentally and emotionally draining.

Send a Group Message

What I usually suggest, particularly at this early point, is to find a way to communicate your status in a group fashion with all but those closest to you. The easiest way is to send a group text or email. You might be tempted to do it over social media, but keep in mind that anything you put up on Facebook, Instagram, or any other platform will in most cases always be there. Anytime people look you up, they may have access to it. An email or text is easier to control in terms of who sees it.

The group message can be very simple, something along the lines of this:

I have been diagnosed with cancer and am still undergoing tests. The information at this point is vague, but I'll give you all an update later on when I know more. I'm not sure if I will contact people individually in the future, or if this will be the easiest mode to continue communicating. I'm very grateful for and appreciative of your concern, but please give me and my family some time to take all this in.

Setting boundaries, in a kind way, is very important. But it's also essential that every person and group in your life understand that *their* messages *to you* mean a lot—even if they go unanswered. You can get this point across by including something like this in your text or email:

Please feel free to reach out, but do not be offended if you don't hear back quickly. Your notes and concern mean a tremendous amount to me, but there is so much going on in my life right now that it's hard to respond to every email, text, call, or card. Thank you for understanding.

It's Okay to Delegate

If you don't have the energy to send out these group emails or texts yourself, don't hesitate to ask for help. During the early days of treatment, your partner, your family members, and your closest circle of friends will often feel a sense of helplessness. They can't do anything to *cure* your cancer, but they are desperate to do whatever possible to make your life easier. So soliciting their assistance at this stage can serve two purposes: It helps make them feel useful, and it gets the word out quicker about your situation.

If possible, divide up the tasks. Maybe a colleague can take care of contacting people at work, a close friend can do the same with that group, and a sibling or cousin can handle your distant relatives or (if applicable) the parents of your children's friends. While the bulk of the message can be the same, it's a good idea to tweak it a bit for each group, depending on what you feel comfortable sharing. You may, for instance, want to include certain details with your extended family but not with your work friends.

Explaining Cancer to Children

If you are recently diagnosed and have children, or live with children to whom you are close, your initial protective impulse may be to not tell them about your cancer. While these feelings are understandable, children are quite perceptive and will likely realize there is a change in the household. They may overhear conversations, and could become confused by the snippets they pick up. As a result, they might think that the situation is worse than it actually is—but because they are afraid to ask, they will be left isolated with their silent concerns.

This is a time to build trust and model open communication. Even children as young as two or three years old will notice a difference whether you tell them or not, as I did when my mother was diagnosed with cancer. So I am speaking from professional and personal experience when I say it's better to be open with kids. Of course, I understand every family is different, and you know your situation best.

Use the Word "Cancer" with Kids

If you use the word "sick" or "illness," like you do when someone has a cold or the flu, children—especially younger children—may automatically generalize and think that *any* illness they might get could be just like what you're going through with cancer. There are entire books written about this topic, some of which are listed in the resources at the end of this book.

Here are some general suggestions you may want to consider when sharing your cancer diagnosis with children of any age, understanding, of course, that you know your kids best. (After this section, you'll find additional age-specific guidance.)

- Pick a time to speak when you (and whoever else is present) are not rushed. If you have multiple children at different ages/ developmental stages, you may want to have separate conversations with each of them.
- Provide information simply and clearly, appropriate to the child's age/developmental level (see following sections).
- Consider practicing ahead of time what you want to say.
- Reassure them that they did not cause the cancer.
- Emphasize that cancer is not contagious.

- Explain that you may sometimes feel different due to the treatment, *not* the cancer itself. Give examples, such as being tired or sleepy after chemotherapy infusions.
- Reiterate to them that if you are emotionally distraught, or feeling unwell physically, they are *not* to blame.
- Maintain a family calendar for all to see, with your treatment days clearly marked. That way they know ahead of time what to expect, and can prepare for when you may not feel so well.
- Ask them open-ended questions—those you can't answer with a simple "yes" or "no"—to gauge their level of understanding, such as, "Can you explain to me what I just said about the cancer?"
- Reassure them that they are loved, and let them know they can still hug and cuddle with you—it won't hurt you. If that ever changes, it will be due to the treatment, and you will tell them ahead of time if possible.
- Provide the opportunity for them to ask questions, and let them know they can always do so in the future. If they don't ask anything right away, check back periodically.
- Don't hesitate to express your own feelings. By showing emotion, you will provide a healthy model that gives children permission to do the same.
- If they ask, "Are you going to die?" consider saying something like, "I hope not (or don't expect to). That is why I am doing this treatment. I will fight to get well. I want to be here with you."
- Notify their schools and others involved with the children about your health situation.
- Keep the same routine as much as possible.
- Use the same caregivers whenever you can.
- If anxiety, depression, or behavioral problems interfere with the child's daily functioning, seek mental health support for them. Sometimes teachers are the first to notice behavioral and emotional changes.

Children Five and Under

For children five years old and under, try to:

- Keep your conversations present focused, on the here and now.
- Teach them words they can use to express their feelings.
- If they can't use words, see if they can share their feelings through drawing or play.
- Encourage them to engage in physical activities.
- If you are in the hospital, or away, have regular video chats with them.

Patient Voices

*"My son is four and knows that I take medicine each day.
I break information into small, palatable chunks that directly
relate to him. The medicine sometimes makes me tired or
sick to my stomach, but it is making me stronger each day so
I can keep playing with him. This feels like the right balance
of being open and honest while still protecting his innocence
and joy in the moment." —Amber M.*

Children Ages Six to Twelve

For children ages six to twelve years old (chronologically or developmentally), you may also consider that:

- Different children have different needs for information. Some want a lot, and others not as much. You know your kids best, so do what feels right.
- Children in this age range may want to look up information on the Internet, so do your best to monitor and oversee their usage.
- The Internet is *not* the best resource because the information is too general and already outdated. Explain to them that every cancer/treatment is different; this is especially important if

they know people who have died of cancer. Ask and encourage them to come to you with questions.

- Assure them that it is still okay to have fun when an adult in their life has cancer. Let them know they can enjoy themselves with their friends and be active in and out of school, even if you are not feeling well.

Teenagers

For teenagers, here are some additional things to keep in mind:

- Teenagers' way of thinking allows for more of a focus on the future, so the conversation can be more complicated. Be prepared to answer lots of "what-if" and "when" questions.
- Include teens in your decision-making where appropriate. For example, ask them who at their schools should be informed about your condition.
- Reiterate to them that every cancer is different, even within a particular *type* of cancer (different lymphomas, leukemias, breast cancers, etc.), and that your treatment is specific for *your cancer*. Remind them that the Internet is not the best source of information because of these nuances.
- Offer to allow them to speak with your healthcare team, if appropriate.
- Teenagers are typically trying to separate and form their own individual identities, so your cancer complicates this developmental stage for them. Try to be understanding, and not take any anger or moodiness as a sign they don't care.
- Some teens will act out because of the situation, while others will keep feelings in so as not to worry you.
- Honesty remains the best policy; be as truthful as possible when teens ask for information.
- Some teens want to be *too* helpful. Encourage them to still go out, have fun, and enjoy themselves with their friends.

- Look into possible support groups or peer support for them. Your hospital may have (or know about) programs designed for teens whose parents/grandparents have cancer.

Sharing Ongoing Updates and Rallying the Troops

Beyond the initial sharing of news, you'll likely want to keep the adults in your life updated as the days and weeks pass. Here are a few ways of managing these ongoing communications.

Nonprofit Health Platforms

A great interactive method of keeping people updated on your health status—and ways that they can help you if they so desire—is by setting up a free, private website through a nonprofit health platform such as *CaringBridge* or *Lotsa Helping Hands*. These sites are designed specifically for this purpose and can be easily updated on a regular basis as your treatment situation and needs change. Anyone interested in how you are doing or how they can help can check in through a dedicated URL, without feeling they are bothering you. You can include photos with your posts, and if you think you might need help running your site, this would be a great job for one or more of your tech-savvy family members or friends.

Here are some examples of posts you (or your proxy) could put up on such a website:

- *Just got home from chemotherapy infusion No. 1. Can't thank the great staff at Dana-Farber enough for making the experience as comfortable as possible. I even got a free hand massage from a massage therapist!*
- *John is going to the hospital for chemo every three weeks and needs help getting his kids rides to and from school on dates X, Y, and Z. Here's a chart listing all their schedules. Please consider taking an AM or PM slot by filling in your name, and thank you in advance.*

- *I'm still wiped out two days after chemo and can't go in to work today. I'd like to try and catch up at home over the weekend, so I've had a small bag of files left for me at the front desk of my office. If somebody can pick the bag up and drop it off at my house, please text me and I'll let them know you're coming. Thanks so much!*

Young adults especially appreciate being told ways they can help, because, as we've already discussed, most of them have never gone through something like cancer. In addition, they are often so busy with their own lives that they may not be fully aware of all you're dealing with at any given time. Providing them with specific ideas of how to be helpful and options like these alleviates a lot of the uncertainty.

Emails/Texts

If you don't want to go the private website route, your group texts or emails can also serve as a way of gently asking for additional help through a line at the end like *No pressure, of course, but if you have time to consider them, here are some suggestions of things that could be helpful to me.*

Social Media

You can also, of course, post status updates or ask for help on social media. This is especially tempting because it's so easy; you just type something up quickly, attach a photo if you so desire, and it's done—you don't have to worry about tailoring a post to different groups or whether you left anybody out.

This approach is fine, but just keep in mind what I warned about earlier—social media posts have long shelf lives. In five, ten, or fifteen years, when you might be looking for a new job or exploring the online dating world, someone could come across posts about your first chemotherapy infusion or the day you decided to shave off your remaining hair.

I'm not implying you should *hide* your cancer treatment from a prospective boss or romantic partner, but you might want the option of telling them yourself rather than having them learn about it on social media. If that's a concern, consider one of the more controllable options.

Dealing with People You Did—and Did *Not*—Expect to Hear From

Don't be surprised in the early stages of treatment if you start getting emails and texts from people you have not heard from in years. Cancer news tends to travel quickly, and those you share it with might wind up spreading that information to others in your wider circle of friends, former colleagues and classmates, and distant relatives.

If you're getting people coming out of the woodwork like this, it might be best to use the same all-at-once strategy that you used to share news of your diagnosis. Rather than responding directly to each note, forward them to whoever is helping with your group messages and have these new well-wishers added to the appropriate list of friends, colleagues, or family.

One disappointing surprise you may encounter is that some folks who you would *expect* to hear from will wind up *not* checking in. Patients tell me all the time about people that they really thought would come through for them with kind words and help, but then either never reached out or broke off contact after one note. This can be very, very painful, but try and focus your energy for now on all those who *are* there for you. (In Chapter 8, we will discuss "cancer ghosting.")

Who Makes Up a Cancer-Treatment Team?

As you begin looking ahead to your cancer-treatment plan, whatever that might be, you'll learn quickly that you won't be interacting with just one doctor, as you might be used to when seeing your primary care physician (PCP) or specialists in other areas like GI or dermatology. Instead, there will be an entire *team* of doctors, nurses, and other clinicians and support staff working together to help you. If you're not sure whether any of these providers are available at a particular treatment center, ask; in some cases, even if they are not on-site, they may be available on an as-needed basis.

Oncologists

First up, you'll meet an oncologist, who you were probably referred to for further tests and diagnosis by your PCP or another clinician. It's important to keep in mind, however, that while the term "oncology" refers to the entire area of medicine dealing with cancer, there are different physician specialists *within* oncology—all of whom have completed college, medical school, and a residency. These include:

- **Surgical oncologists**, who have general surgical training and a specialty fellowship in cancer surgery
- **Radiation oncologists**, who possess specialized training in using radiation to treat cancer
- **Medical oncologists**, who complete an internal medicine residency and a fellowship in oncology
- **Hematologic oncologists**, who specialize in treating cancers of the blood, like leukemia

In many cases, the medical oncologist coordinates all the care among the different members of your clinical team. For example, the medical oncologist will refer you to the surgical oncologist if surgery is being considered, or the radiation oncologist if that treatment is a possibility.

Other Important Team Members

Other key team members are nurses, nurse practitioners (commonly called NPs), physician assistants (PAs), and medical assistants (MAs). All these healthcare professionals provide very important aspects of your care. Often you will initially see your medical oncologist and/or surgical oncologist to discuss your overall treatment plan, and then on follow-up visits meet with the PA or NP. MAs will usually take your blood pressure and vital signs when you arrive for appointments, while nurses generally administer chemotherapy during your infusions.

If you are treated at an academic cancer center—one affiliated with a medical school, like Dana-Farber is with Harvard Medical School—you'll likely also have trainees on your team including both residents (trainees who completed medical school) and fellows, those who have finished residency and are now doing fellowships (specialized training) in surgical oncology, medical oncology, or radiation oncology. Different types of trainees may also be on hand during each stage of treatment, observing and learning.

Radiation Oncology

About 50 to 60 percent of cancer patients will undergo radiation therapy. If radiation is needed, a separate team headed up by the radiation oncologist becomes involved to make sure that this powerful, targeted treatment is administered safely and accurately. Radiation therapists will actually administer your radiation treatments, which usually occur daily for several weeks (with weekends off).

Palliative Care Team

Many people associate the term "palliative care" with end-of-life care, but that's not necessarily the case. They are not synonyms. As an area of medicine, palliative care is focused on treating pain, managing symptoms, and maintaining quality of life *throughout* your cancer journey, starting at diagnosis. Research has highlighted the benefits of this practice. One seminal study showed that lung cancer patients who received palliative care from the time of their diagnosis not only experienced better management of their cancer and treatment-related symptoms than lung cancer patients who lacked this support, they also *lived longer*. So if you are dealing with multiple symptoms that are interfering with your ability to live your best possible life, you definitely want palliative care involved—and the earlier the better.

Additional Specialists

Depending on the type and stage of your cancer, and where you are treated, there are other clinicians who might become part of your team. If you've had certain kinds of surgery, such as a mastectomy for breast cancer or head and neck cancer surgery, reconstructive surgeons may work with your surgical oncologist. Integrative medicine specialists can offer you acupuncture, massage, or other approaches to help with quality of life during treatment. Mental health professionals including social workers, psychiatrists, and psychologists (like myself) might also be a vital part of your team, and we will discuss their roles later on.

Talking to Your Treatment Team about Supplements and Recreational Drug Use

Even under "normal" conditions, most people are reluctant to share with healthcare providers about their use of alcohol, recreational drugs, and dietary or other supplements. However, given the seriousness of the treatment you're about to undergo, it's imperative that you overcome that hesitancy and be open and honest about what you're currently using (or considering). Don't worry about judgment—your health is the most important thing on your care team's minds, and it's important they have a complete list of what's entering your body to make the most educated decisions possible about treatment.

Vitamins and Supplements

We've already discussed how people you have not heard from in years will likely begin reaching out after your diagnosis. Don't be surprised if some of them mention vitamins, supplements, and herbs and insist you start taking them *immediately* to deal with your cancer. Trying to be helpful, they will tell you things like, "I know this guy who took shark cartilage, or megadoses of vitamin C, and it was really helpful."

If this happens to you, whether or not you've already listened to such suggestions, it is vital that you tell your oncologist or someone on your oncology team. Be open and honest: "I have been taking (or considering taking) X, Y, and Z, and I want to know if there is a possibility that some of them could interfere with my cancer treatment." You should not be embarrassed to ask these questions, and it's critically important that you *do* ask them. Even if your oncologist does not know the answers, most academic medical centers will have integrative medicine specialists who can work with the oncology team to provide appropriate guidance.

Recreational Drug Use

Another thing you should be open about discussing before starting treatment—without fear of judgment—is if you are currently using any type of recreational drugs. It is widely understood that young adulthood is a stage of life when people experiment and try new things, so don't worry what your oncology team will think of you. It's important that you tell them about any drugs you are taking, so *they* can tell *you* of any possible negative interactions with your cancer treatment. If you are taking cannabis recreationally—whether by smoking, edibles, or oils—there may be the possibility of your continuing to take it for medicinal use. You won't know, however, if you don't discuss it.

The same goes for tobacco products. If you are smoking, chewing, or vaping, don't be worried about admitting this to your oncology team. Remember, there is no stigma in an oncology center! You need to share that information. Maybe you are doing cocaine, or since you were diagnosed someone has suggested you try some psychedelic mushrooms recreationally to help you cope. Whatever it is, you need to communicate with your team and let them provide you with guidance. There are even specialists at many cancer centers who your oncologist can connect you with to discuss other drug/medication options that are safe to take during treatment.

Key Points

- Sharing your initial diagnosis and subsequent health updates with people in your life can be draining and overwhelming. Consider delegating this task to loved ones who want to help.
- Talking to kids about cancer can feel uncomfortable, but being honest is usually the best course. You can still use age-appropriate language and approaches while being open and answering questions.
- You'll be working with a team of people during your treatment and care. These healthcare professionals will help guide you throughout one of the most difficult and complicated challenges you will ever face, so it's critically important to understand their different roles.
- It's also imperative to be transparent with your treatment team, even about awkward topics. If you are taking or considering vitamins, supplements, or recreational drugs, be sure to tell them.

CHAPTER 4

Coping with Cancer Treatment

Matt was twenty-six, working in sales at a department store, when he noticed a cut on his tongue one day during his lunch break. Although surprised it didn't heal quickly, he didn't give it much thought.

A few months later, Matt's dentist observed the still-unhealed cut during a routine checkup and referred him to a head and neck surgeon for a workup. The results of the biopsy came back as tongue cancer.

"I was shocked because I had always heard that mouth cancer was associated with tobacco and alcohol use," Matt recalls. "I never smoked, chewed, or drank, and had only tried pot a few times back in high school."

Told he needed surgery to remove a portion of his tongue, Matt was worried about how it would affect his appearance—and his ability to speak and perform his job. Those fears only grew after the procedure. His mouth hurt tremendously, he struggled with pronunciation, and he thought the stitches on his neck made him look like something out of a horror movie. While on leave from work to recover, he seldom left his apartment.

The surgeon encouraged Matt to be patient and give it a couple of months. He was referred to a speech therapist to help with swallowing and talking, and also met with an oncology dietitian, who provided a nutrition plan. Matt's brother temporarily moved in to help out.

"My boyfriend visited me every day, and he and my brother were both very supportive," Matt explains. "But I was pissed off having to repeat myself all the time because I couldn't pronounce certain words, and took out my frustration on both of them."

Matt felt depressed and scared. He lost weight, tired easily, and wondered if he would ever have the strength, stamina, and language skills needed to resume his routine of nine-hour days on his feet talking to customers.

"When my medical team referred me to a psychologist who worked with head and neck patients, that really helped," recalls Matt. "She encouraged me to tell her the improvements I had noticed those first eight weeks, and as I did I realized how much better my speech had gotten—and that my scar was healing."

The psychologist and a dietitian teamed up to make sure Matt got the calories he needed, and after he started taking daily walks, his weight and endurance gradually came back. One big fear was not being able to kiss his boyfriend again, but with speech therapy, Matt gradually relearned to do that as well.

"There were still moments every day when I would get upset," Matt admits. "But I kept reminding myself how much progress I was making, and tried to stay focused on the tasks at hand."

Putting Your Blinders On (for Now)

Part of what makes cancer challenging is that it is not just *one* threatening situation. Rather, it is a series of crises that make up your cancer trajectory. Some are anticipated, like starting a new phase of treatment—say, switching from chemotherapy to radiation. Other times, though, the threat is unexpected—such as an allergic reaction to a new chemo drug or an infection due to low white blood cell counts.

Here's some encouraging news: Usually, once your active treatment starts, your focus will be directed on getting through each stage of it. You may still fear for your survival, but you are no longer in that constant fight-or-flight state. Think of it as putting your blinders on—in a good way.

Your mind will be on the treatment, the side effects, and the impact they will have on your life in terms of disruptions and interruptions. Assuming you get a well-prescribed course of therapy, you can try to compartmentalize and say, "This is now my focus." As feelings come up, you can deal with them. But if things go pretty smoothly, you can keep those blinders on and plow right through. Bigger existential questions—like what it all *means* to you, and to your future—may be put on hold until the end of treatment. We will address those in later chapters.

Putting your blinders on goes a long way, but you should still be aware of what lies ahead. While this is not a medical textbook, a review of the main cancer treatments and their common side effects—along with coping strategies for each—will give you a solid foundation of knowledge. This chapter will focus largely on surgery, radiation, and chemotherapy and also take a brief look at targeted therapies and immunotherapies. Once you have a clearer understanding of them all, you will be better poised to ask questions of your healthcare team and help to shape your treatment plan.

Surgery

Surgery is essentially the process of removing the cancer tumor(s) from your body. There is lots of variability in terms of what to expect from surgery, depending on the extent of the procedure, the type of cancer you have, and its location. Different surgeries will also result in different potential side effects, as well as varying rehabilitation options and recovery time frames.

Even if your surgery is not huge, per se, it is still cancer surgery. It is that diagnosis and what it *means* that is so frightening. A part of your body is going to be changed in some way, and that can be a threat to your sense of your body integrity. This thought is more troubling for some people than others, and certain cancer surgeries may have a greater emotional impact on individuals. Remember, just like with a cancer diagnosis, there is no "right" or "wrong" way to feel about surgery. They are your feelings, and that is what's important.

Goals of Cancer Surgery

The usual goal for cancer surgery is to remove all or most of your tumor(s) while still considering cosmetic and functional outcomes. No matter which surgery you have, you want a surgeon who is both trained in oncology (called a surgical oncologist) and has additional expertise in your specific procedure. For instance, surgical oncologists with proficiency in head and neck surgeries are skilled at trying to work along the natural lines of your neck or face, and they may involve a plastic/reconstructive surgeon to ensure things look as natural as possible.

Surgery Choices, Reconstructive Options, and Rehab

At times you may have surgical options. With early stage breast cancer, for example, you may be able to opt for a lumpectomy (removing just the tumor) or a mastectomy (removing most of the breast). Trying to make a choice can feel overwhelming. Speaking with a mental health professional trained to aid patients in treatment decision-making can help in reviewing and choosing the best option for you. Other times, if circumstances are such that, for instance, a lumpectomy is *not* an option, you can then focus on reconstructive and rehabilitative options—and making *those* choices.

If you decide or need to have reconstructive surgery, you want a plastic surgeon who specializes in reconstructive surgery, specifically on the part of your body impacted by the cancer. You should also ask them specific questions, like:

- How many reconstructions like this have you done?
- Can I see some before-and-after pictures of patients who have had the surgery?
- Can I speak with patients who have had it?
- If I am not ready to do reconstructive surgery now, can I still get it later?

Remember, just because you have the option for reconstructive surgery does not mean you have to get it. For example, some patients decide to use a prosthesis instead of undergoing breast reconstruction, while some use nothing and get a tattoo to cover their chest. Still other patients may not be ready right away to make a decision about reconstruction.

After testicular surgery, some men opt for a testicular prosthesis—since usually just one of their two testes is removed. Others may not feel they want the prosthesis, then later change their minds and get it. Some women get immediate breast reconstruction, while others wait.

In terms of rehabilitation, you may want to prepare questions to help you plan ahead and line up the resources you will need. Health-care teams do focus on rehabilitative options, but depending where you get your treatment, some of these referrals may not be as well integrated into your overall care. This section will give you some examples and suggestions for options you may need to directly inquire about, depending on the surgery—including speech therapy, swallowing therapy, physical therapy, pelvic floor physical therapy, occupational therapy, and pulmonary rehabilitation. Support from a mental health provider familiar with your treatment may also help you in finding ways to deal with side effects, problem-solve solutions and work-arounds, and connect with resources.

Handling Functional Impairments

Most young adults are accustomed to being able to rely on their bodies to function "normally" with little thought to what could change that. After surgery, however, you might find yourself facing "functional impairments"—which is a fancy way of saying "your body can't yet perform all the usual daily tasks at the degree to which you are accustomed." Asking questions early on can help alleviate concerns about functional changes.

Speaking, Eating, and Drinking

Functional impairments are particularly daunting when they involve very basic skills, such as speaking, eating, and drinking. These impairments are common after head and neck surgeries, like the challenges that Matt from the start of the chapter faced. Keep in mind, however, that many of your speech and swallowing difficulties will be temporary. Getting speech therapy and swallowing therapy to help you regain your ability to speak, eat, and swallow is critically important.

This therapy takes time, and it may help to plan ahead and be ready for different scenarios—such as going through a drive-through window, making phone calls, or joining friends for dinner. I routinely work with patients to develop their own phrases to have at the ready so they are prepared to respond when approaching new situations that may require answering or asking questions.

Breathing

Lung cancer surgery can also be extremely difficult, because it may result in a change in your breathing that leaves you short of breath at times—particularly after you've exerted yourself. You will need to learn to slow down and take breaks, even if that means not being able to keep up with your peers on hikes, the basketball court, or vacations. This can present a challenge socially, and also be very embarrassing to talk about. Sharing your circumstances with others can help you break the ice and ease your mind. Pulmonary rehabilitation is an option, and while not all institutions offer this, ask your healthcare team if a referral is appropriate.

Bowel Changes

When it comes to GI cancers, such as colorectal, the type of surgery you have will depend on the location and extent of your tumor. Accordingly, the side effects and functional impairments that may result from surgery vary, and can be either temporary or more permanent. One thing you might experience right after surgery are bowel changes, including more frequent bowel movements and a change in consistency. You may feel a need to go to the bathroom more often, a sensation known as urgency, or have some difficulty with controlling your bowels. Such control is one of those bodily functions people often take for granted, and any change in it can impact your ability to leave home without worrying. This may also occur with some gynecological surgeries. Make sure you ask your healthcare team for medications to help manage these usually temporary side effects. Pelvic floor physical therapy can also provide assistance with urgency and bowel control. If you need help in this area, ask for a prescription and referral to a physical therapist with this training. Peer mentors can be an invaluable resource in suggesting ways to cope.

Physical Movement

Your ability to move might also be affected by surgery. For example, with sarcomas (cancers of the connective tissues such as bones, fat, and muscles), there can be some post-surgery functional impairment depending on the location and type of procedure you have. Today care teams really try to minimize your surgery to avoid functional impairments, and it's important to see a rehab physician after whatever procedure you have done. Based on their recommendations, you may also need to get physical therapy and/or occupational therapy.

Sexual Function

Changes to sexual abilities also fall under functional impairment, and it's important to get all the facts rather than make assumptions. For example, testicular cancer does not usually have any impact on your ability to have an erection and ejaculate, but you won't know if you don't ask.

Post-Op Body Image

Some surgeries have a more noticeable impact on parts of your body that are visible to others around you. Head and neck surgeries, for example, can leave swelling and scars that are not as easily hidden as the effects from other procedures. For young people who are still developing their body images, this situation can be very challenging. You may seek out ways to avoid the scrutiny. My mother, whose cancer journey I'll discuss more later, temporarily wore scarves after having a radical neck dissection at age twenty-seven. This kept her from needing to explain the scar on her neck from the surgery.

Radiation Therapy

Radiation therapy involves delivering radiation to a specific part of your body where cancer is/was located. This is done in a very focused and targeted fashion so it causes the least damage possible to other areas around the cancerous region. Great advances have been made in recent years to the radiation process, making it more precise than ever.

Length of Radiation

Radiation often lasts several weeks. The exact length of time depends on the specifics of your cancer, but usually treatments run from Monday through Friday. This can seem like an overwhelming time commitment, but keep in mind that the actual treatments are very brief—just a few minutes each day. In fact, from the moment you check in, change into a gown, get placed on the radiation table, receive your treatment, and then put your clothes back on, the whole session takes about thirty minutes. So while it *is* daily, it's at the same time each day, and you get in and out pretty quickly. You can also ask to listen to your favorite music while you are inside the radiation suite to help distract you.

Side Effects of Radiation

Depending on your specific cancer, the location of the tumor being radiated, the type of radiation you are receiving, and the dosage of the radiation, different side effects can occur.

What to Ask Your Doctor

Given the variability of possible side effects from radiation, asking some of the following questions may be of assistance so you can anticipate challenges and put a plan of action in place before commencing radiation treatment:

- How will my skin change, and what will the changes look like?
- When will I first notice the changes?
- Are they temporary or permanent?
- What can I do to help prevent or heal the skin changes?
- Should I avoid sun on the area receiving radiation?
- Do most patients experience burning and pain from treatment in this area? How long does such pain last?

- What do you do to treat the pain? Do you have a pain-management/palliative care team who could prescribe topical relief or other pain management?
- Will my hair thin or fall out completely in the area receiving radiation? Is it temporary or permanent?
- What other side effect(s) do you anticipate I might have and what will you do to help with them?

How Long Side Effects Last

It's very important to remember that as difficult as these reactions can seem at the time, they are often temporary—they will go away in the weeks after your radiation is completed. If your radiation is for five to six weeks, most side effects will usually start to emerge after two to three weeks into your treatment and continue for two to four additional weeks after it's completed. Remember that radiation therapy is a localized treatment, and any side effects—with the exception of fatigue—are associated with the part of your body being treated. Medical teams often underestimate recovery time, which can lead to understandable surprise and frustration around why patients don't feel "back to normal" immediately after completing radiation. Try to be patient and compassionate with yourself.

Fatigue

Fatigue is common regardless of type, dosage, and location of radiation treatment. Given your age, thinking about how to allocate your energy is probably not something you've really had to concern yourself with until now. Try to give yourself several months after treatment completion before expecting your energy level to bounce back. Later in this chapter, we will address ways to cope with treatment-related fatigue, which is one of the most disruptive side effects for young adults.

Chemotherapy

Chemotherapy is often what people most associate with being a cancer patient. It is also probably the most feared portion of treatment, due in large part, I believe, to what it was like in the past—as well as the imagery we still see portrayed in movies and television shows.

Many patients have shared with me that they felt they could have largely kept their cancer private if they'd just had surgery, although it's more difficult if the effects of surgery are extremely visible. Chemotherapy, on the other hand, is what makes the cancer feel *real* and *public* for many. The regular outpatient trips to the hospital for infusions, as well as the resulting fatigue, hair loss, and other side effects, make cancer a regular part of your calendar and your life.

People have lots of varying feelings, some of them influenced in part by their cultural backgrounds, about how much they want to share their cancer with the outside world during this period. If you have children, however, you may want to be more transparent. Create and display a calendar for your chemotherapy infusions and other treatments so your kids know the days you may not feel well or be as interactive with them. This will help them understand that it is the chemo making you not feel well—it is not their fault, and has nothing to do with their behavior. While your family's routine may be different on certain days as visible on the calendar, keep reminding them that it's *not* a permanent change.

Prepping for Chemo with a Port

Before starting chemotherapy, your clinical team may recommend that you get a specific type of portacath (or "port"). This device reduces the need for you to have repeated needle sticks to your arm each time someone on your team needs to access one of your veins for a blood draw or chemotherapy infusion or to give you fluids or antibiotics. The port is implanted under your skin, on your upper chest, in a very short procedure done under general anesthesia. It consists of a catheter that is attached internally to one of your veins, and a small, rounded basin at the top about the size of a quarter. You can feel the basin under your skin, but it's usually not visible to others.

You may not be thrilled with the idea of having something foreign inside your body, but there are many benefits to getting a port. It can be accessed easily with one needle stick, and a tube attached to the needle allows your team to handle all of your blood draws, infusions, and other needs for an entire day of treatment. There is nothing you need to worry about cleaning or taking out at home. If you feel discomfort the first time your port is being accessed, you can ask to have lidocaine sprayed over it on future visits to numb the area before the needle stick. Besides being more convenient, a port helps to prevent scarring and damage to your veins from repeated needle sticks, which makes accessing the veins more difficult.

Yes, a port is *another* change to your body and your appearance. Even if it is not very visible, you know it's there. For some people, it's a constant reminder that they are going through cancer treatment, especially if they have less fat around their chest area—making the indentation of the port's basin more noticeable through their skin. Your clinical team may also ask you to restrict some of your body movements to prevent your port from becoming dislocated, and there is the rare possibility of getting an infection or blood clot from the device.

Still, despite these challenges, I believe a port is definitely worth it. It makes one of the most annoying and stressful parts of cancer a lot easier, and it can stay safely in for as long as you need it. Then, once you have completed treatment, it can be removed in a quick outpatient procedure.

Getting Through Chemo

This section will walk you through a typical chemo cycle, so you know both what to expect and what *not* to worry about—especially if you've seen some of those movie scenes.

Day One

Let's call each time you come in for an infusion Day One of that chemo cycle. As you might expect, the day of your first infusion is always the scariest due to fear of the unknown. No matter how much people try to prepare you for it, chemo is probably unlike anything you've gone through. And, as we've discussed in earlier chapters, some patients can get so anxious that they experience nausea or diarrhea before their treatment even starts. If this happens to you, and your stress level is so high in the days leading up to your first infusion that it's interfering with your functioning or even your ability to sleep, talk to your treatment team about taking an oral antianxiety medication before coming in on the mornings of your treatments. That way you can start each cycle in a more relaxed place.

Because of the premedications that patients now receive in their IVs right before chemotherapy, you will likely actually feel pretty good the day of your infusions. These medications help prevent nausea and vomiting and improve how you feel in general—and are a pleasant surprise to lots of people.

Another surprise is that you may feel hungry when done with your infusions—or even *during* them. At Dana-Farber, we have volunteers who hand out sandwiches and snacks to people undergoing infusions. If you don't feel like eating then, you may be up for lunch or dinner out after you leave. Most people feel pretty good energy-wise on Day One due to the premedications, except perhaps after their first treatment—when the tension surrounding this new experience can be especially exhausting.

Once you've gotten your first Day One under your belt, you will likely find the treatments become easier because you know what to expect.

Day Two and Beyond

You will probably still feel pretty good at the beginning of the day after each infusion, or Day Two. Toward the *end* of Day Two or beginning of Day Three, however, a general feeling of malaise will often start to set in. Your body will ache, and the fatigue will grow. You'll also likely lose your appetite. These feelings will typically last anywhere from Day Two/Three to Day Five, and for some people even a whole week (up to Day Seven or Day Eight). There is some variability, depending on the chemo regimen that you're on. Make sure you take all of the medications prescribed by your oncology team, especially those to prevent nausea and vomiting.

Things will then gradually improve, at least in terms of how your body feels, until your next infusion. Your white blood cell counts may decrease seven to fourteen days after treatment, which could increase your risk of infection. Your team will monitor you at follow-up visits during this period, and let you know if you need to take precautions.

Starting the Cycle Again

The first time you go through an entire chemotherapy cycle, just like the lead-up to your first infusion, is the toughest. You may be afraid, and when you begin feeling achy, nauseated, and fatigued, you might think it's never going to end. You might wonder, "How am I going to deal with this every day?"

Once you *have* gone through it once, however, you'll know what to expect. Even though some parts of your cycle may be extremely difficult, you can now be more confident they will pass and you'll have a good week (or a few good weeks) before your next infusion. I will often ask patients to write down or make an audio or video recording of their improvements, and then refer to it later to help remind themselves that the bad feelings will pass. Experience, in this case, is a form of medicine.

Side Effects from Chemo

Cancer cells tend to divide quickly. Chemotherapy is designed to target these rapidly dividing cells, and damages them at the different stages of cell replication. In a sense, chemo attempts to kill the cancer cells. Unfortunately, it often also impacts *other* quickly dividing cells in our bodies—such as hair follicles, bone marrow, and the linings of the gastrointestinal system. This is what leads to side effects. The following are some common side effects resulting from chemotherapy, and suggestions for dealing with them.

Hair Loss

This is the side effect that the public most associates with chemotherapy, and cancer treatment in general, because it's so visible. Not *all* chemotherapies result in hair loss; depending on the chemo you get, your hair may thin rather than fall out, or you may not lose it at all.

If you do lose your hair (a process called alopecia), this will usually begin two to three weeks into your chemotherapy treatment. How will you know when your hair starts falling out? Believe me, you will definitely know. You will put your hand to your head, and strands will sprinkle down. You will lie on a pillow, and the pillow will suddenly be full of hair. It will come off in your comb or hairbrush and go down the drain when you're showering.

Hair loss can dramatically impact your emotional well-being. You look in the mirror, and the change is right there staring back at you. Hair means different things to different people, but generally within American society, hair symbolizes youth, vitality, and health. Even though you have not aged, that symbol of your youth feels gone. Unless you are already balding naturally, or have previously shaved your head, people may not initially recognize you. You might not even recognize *yourself*. It's completely normal to wind up being very upset by this. People may say not to worry, because the hair loss is temporary, but it's a loss nonetheless—and you are entitled to your feelings.

Ideas for Dealing with Hair Loss

How you deal with hair loss really depends on what you feel most comfortable with. There is no right or wrong way, whether you let your hair fall out as the treatment dictates, shave your head immediately upon noticing any hair loss, or try something else. Here are a few ideas:

- If you have longer hair, you could transition slowly. Cut some off, get adjusted to a shorter length, and then shave it off completely once your hair really starts to fall out.
- If your hair begins coming out in patches, use scalp concealers (which are inexpensive and easy to use) to fill in some of the bald spots. Then, once you can no longer cover the missing patches, shave it all off.

- Take charge by shaving your hair off "live" at a party with friends. Maybe some friends can shave theirs, too, as a sign of solidarity. This idea is not for everyone, but it can be a really meaningful memory.
- If you are getting a wig, try to do so *before* you lose your hair—so you are ready when it happens. Some people opt for a wig that looks exactly like their hair texture, color, and cut. Nobody except those they tell will even know they've lost their hair. Others use this opportunity to try a new color, texture, and/or style. Ask your medical team for a list of referrals for wig shops accustomed to dealing with alopecia.
- Wigs can be expensive, but insurance may cover some or all of the costs. Get a prescription from your oncology team for a hair prosthesis, and submit it to your insurance.
- Not everyone wants a natural-hair wig, which is the most expensive type and requires more upkeep. Ask to see all types of wigs before making your decision. Take a friend or family member to help you choose, and advocate for your choice. A list of free wig organizations for those who qualify financially is in the Resources section of this book.
- If you're feeling adventurous, buy several inexpensive wigs in a wild array of colors and styles to wear on different occasions.
- Wigs can get itchy and uncomfortable after a full day of wear, especially in hot weather. You may want to buy a few hats and caps as another option. Some, designed specifically for people dealing with hair loss, have ponytails and/or bangs sewn into them.
- Scarves, on their own or under a hat, can provide bursts of color and a way to help express your personality. Be sure to get cotton scarves—silk scarves will slide off your head easily.
- At home, and even out and about, you may find it easier and more comfortable to wear soft turbans or nothing at all. Remember, you don't *have* to cover your head if you don't want to do so.

- Instead of wearing wigs or hats, get a temporary henna tattoo on your head.
- If you cut off at least 10 inches of your hair (tip to tip), you can bundle it into a ponytail or braid and donate it to Locks of Love, a charity that creates prosthetic hairpieces for children dealing with medically related hair loss.

Explaining Hair Loss to Kids

If you have young children, or share a home with them, it's important to prepare them for your hair loss. It is unlikely that you're going to want to wear a wig or scarf all the time, particularly in your home—where you'll want the chance to relax and feel more comfortable. So it's better to let them know about the change before they see it for themselves.

Explain that your hair is falling out because you're getting chemotherapy to prevent—or treat—the cancer. Be sure to emphasize that your hair *will* come back. Some of my patients involve their young kids in the process, letting them help cut or shave off their hair. Other people shave privately and then show their children. Even if they are initially upset, most kids will adjust. They often take their cues from you in terms of how to react. If you tear up and cry, it's fine. It gives your children permission to cry themselves. You can always choose to mourn the loss of your hair in private, but having your kids involved is a way to normalize what's happening.

Scalp Cooling

In recent years, a treatment known as scalp cooling has emerged as an option for helping prevent or minimize hair loss during chemotherapy. Scalp cooling involves placing a tight-fitting silicone cap (known as a cold cap) on your head before, during, and after each chemo infusion—a process that reduces blood flow to the cells that produce hair and helps protect them from chemotherapy. You may not be eligible for a cold cap because of your particular type of cancer, or due to your chemotherapy regimen, but if you do qualify, it's worth considering. Ask to see if it's an option. Your insurance may not cover the cost, but some cancer centers have programs to help do so—be sure to inquire. Cold caps can be quite uncomfortable because they are *so* cold they can cause headaches, so they are not for everyone. Maybe consider trying one initially, and if it's too painful, you can stop at any time.

Bald Can Be Beautiful . . . or Not

People tend to think of hair loss as being harder for women. After all, they figure, a lot of men are going to lose their hair at some point, and more young guys than ever today—actors, athletes, even models—are shaving their heads in their twenties and thirties as a fashion statement. But cancer-related hair loss is difficult regardless of your gender. As a young person, if you haven't lost your hair already, going bald when it is not your choice to do so can be devastating. There is a big difference between *choosing* to shave your head and *having* to do so because you're going through chemotherapy.

Other Hair Loss

One thing that may surprise you is that chemo-related hair loss can often happen in other parts of your body. This includes facial hair—such as your eyebrows and lashes—as well as what is often last to go: your pubic hair. There are different ways to deal with these developments, including learning to draw on eyebrows or microblading (a semipermanent form of brow tattooing), but make sure you discuss these with your medical team before trying them.

Nausea (and Conditioned Nausea)

Nausea and vomiting, long-feared side effects of chemotherapy, were once an almost universal problem. These days, because of the very effective anti-nausea regimens that patients receive in their IVs before chemo infusions, it is highly unlikely you will experience any nausea during your actual infusion. You may even, as mentioned before, feel hungry during or right after they are done.

It is important, however, that you follow the recommendations of your team after each chemo infusion. They will give you a particular combination of medications to take at home to prevent nausea and vomiting. If one of these drug regimens doesn't work, let them know—and you can try a different combination.

It is best to treat nausea right away, and prevent it from getting worse, rather than wait. Once it's really bad, it's much harder to get under control. I usually tell patients to use a scale of zero to ten—with zero being no nausea and ten being the worst nausea—and to try and manage their queasiness by keeping it under a five. If it rises above that, it's likely going to be harder to manage.

Unfortunately, due to anxiety, some people still experience nausea *before* their chemotherapy. They may think this feeling is related to the chemo, but it's not, because it actually starts prior to their infusion. Those who have this anxiety-induced nausea are at an increased risk for developing conditioned nausea, in which they associate chemotherapy and the cancer center with feeling nauseated. Once that conditioning kicks in, they will start getting queasy every chemo day—and sometimes even days before it, just by thinking about the upcoming treatment.

Here are some tips if you notice yourself becoming nauseated prior to chemotherapy:

- Immediately ask your team for some antianxiety medication to take at home on the same day as your chemo, before going into the treatment center.
- Have some ginger candy or tea the mornings of your infusions.
- Wear anti-nausea wristbands on chemo days. These target an acupressure point known to help with nausea and are available at most pharmacies.
- Listen to music on the way to treatment and while waiting to get chemo.
- If the cancer center "smell" is what sets you off, try applying a small amount of peppermint or lavender essential oil either

to your wrist or a handkerchief that you bring to treatment. This will distract from the scent you associate with the cancer center—and that may be triggering your nausea.

- Try diaphragmatic breathing before and at the cancer center.
- If these strategies don't work, ask your team for a referral to a psychologist who specializes in treating conditioned nausea/vomiting.

Nutritional Challenges

There is lots of information online about how to eat and drink healthier during cancer treatment, but you need to be cautious before believing what you read. So-called experts will insist there are different herbs and supplements that you *must* take during treatment, and while these folks can be very convincing—and may claim to have all kinds of training—many of the supplements they are pitching are not regulated. You can't even be sure what's in them; some could be harmful to you and perhaps even interfere with your chemotherapy treatment. Check with your team before trying any such wonder supplements.

Dietary Issues

Nutrition is critically important during your treatment, but what you want to eat may be different than usual. Your food preferences during treatment might also change again post-treatment. However tempting, though, this is not the time to start on a new diet or fad. It's important to talk to a registered dietitian (RD) specializing in oncology, who can give you tips to make sure that you're getting the nutrition you need during treatment. An RD can also help you deal with some of the side effects that you may be experiencing.

Nutrition and making sure you eat properly can become a point of contention between you and your partner, family, and/or whomever you are living with. The people in your life all desperately want to help you through your treatment, but they often feel helpless in terms of *what* they can do. As a result, they may look at ensuring you eat and drink healthily, and enough, as one way of being a beneficial part of your treatment and recovery. For this reason, I usually suggest that your family and those who you're living with during your treatment participate in a consultation with an RD. If anyone has concerns about you getting enough nutrition, these can be talked about openly in this group setting.

As with any medical professional, it's important to find an RD who specializes in working with cancer patients—not one primarily focused on helping people lose weight or make lifestyle changes. You need somebody who understands your chemo regimen and toxicity, is familiar with the treatment that you're getting, and can guide you accordingly. Most academic cancer centers will have RDs on staff who are specifically trained in oncology and are knowledgeable in the different nutritional needs around your type of cancer and treatment. For instance, the nutritional plan for breast cancer may be different than the plan needed for head and neck or colorectal cancer.

If you are not being treated at an academic center, look for an RD who is appropriately trained in oncology. RDs have an undergraduate degree and a master's and/or doctorate in the field and have passed a national exam. Some may even have passed another exam to practice in oncology. Dietitians are regulated by each state and are credentialed professionals licensed to provide medical nutrition therapy. Nutritionists are *not* registered dietitians and can have variable training backgrounds and credentials. In many states, they are not regulated either.

Taste Changes

During chemotherapy, you may develop a metallic taste in your mouth, or a lack of taste for certain foods. Some say even water doesn't taste good. This is temporary, and will gradually go away after completing treatment. Miracle fruit, red berries produced by a West African plant, can help you with taste changes. You can buy miracle fruit in some states, or get it in pill form; when you chew the fruit or pill, it actually changes the sour and metallic tastes caused by chemo into something more palatable.

Weight Changes

Some patients lose weight during treatment, while others gain weight. People expect weight loss, and fear "looking like a cancer patient." Weight gain is *not* something you would expect, but part of some chemotherapy treatments for leukemia can include oral steroids—which increase appetite and may cause fluid retention. Early stage breast cancer patients also may gain weight during treatment, likely due to a combination of factors including hormonal changes, activity changes, and pre-treatment steroids. Your muscle mass and tone may also shift.

You might feel very distraught with any fluctuation in weight, because this is an additional attack to your body image and how others react to you. While temporary, it's still difficult and requires reminding yourself things *will* improve after treatment. Your dietitian can provide guidance and tips as well.

Mouth Sores

Another possible chemotherapy side effect is sores inside your mouth, which can be quite painful. Your team might offer to prescribe something for you called "magic mouthwash," which can really help soothe the sores in both your mouth and throat, as well as some oral, topical pain medication. You can also ask your RD to work with you on coming up with nutritional ideas—including fluid nutrition—to further deal with the pain.

Diarrhea

Some chemotherapy regimens can cause diarrhea. Again, it is important to follow the recommendations given to you by your oncology team. If the diarrhea continues, and/or if you're vomiting and become dehydrated, contact your team; you may need to come in for outpatient IV medications and fluids for dehydration.

Cancer-Related Fatigue

Fatigue is the most widely experienced side effect in cancer care. Cancer-related fatigue (CRF) is defined as an overwhelming sense of exhaustion associated with cancer or cancer treatment. It is especially difficult for young adults, who report it as a huge factor in diminished quality of life during treatment. When fatigue is mentioned as a side effect at the start of treatment, you might associate it with a prior time in your life when you felt really tired—and assume that this is the same *type* of tired you'll be experiencing during treatment. But cancer-related fatigue is actually very different from that, and unlike anything you've ever felt before. Rates of CRF vary depending on the type of cancer and treatment you get, and the causes of CRF *during* treatment may be different than those *post*-treatment. (We will cover the latter in a later chapter.)

Finding Patterns and Other Potential Causes

If you are undergoing chemotherapy, during your first treatment cycle you will likely notice when you start to feel an overwhelming sense of fatigue and exhaustion. From this experience, you can anticipate when the same devastating feeling will occur in future chemo cycles. For most people, the sensation does not last the *entire* cycle, but there is somewhat of a cumulative impact. So while you'll experience some post-chemo fatigue for a certain number of days during your first cycle, by the time you get to your *last* one, you may find that the fatigue has accumulated—and you feel even more exhausted. Not until all your treatment is completed will you likely begin gradually recovering your energy.

Other factors can also contribute to CRF. If you're not sleeping well due to worrying, or medications like steroids that keep you up, or aches and unmanaged pain associated with your treatment, that's going to contribute to fatigue, as well as other issues like depression and anxiety. For women used to menstruating regularly, chemotherapy treatment may temporarily put you into premature menopause—which brings its own sleep difficulties due to menopausal symptoms like hot flashes.

A New Challenge

If you're in the early part of young adulthood, say eighteen to thirty, unless you've dealt with a prior serious illness, you've probably never had to think before about conserving your stamina or pacing yourself. You're used to being able to go-go-go from very early in the morning until very late at night, and you may have even pulled some all-nighters while studying or caring for a fussy baby. If you're in your thirties or forties, you've still got the energy needed to juggle the assorted pressures connected to challenges like advancing in your career, paying off your mortgage, and caring for both your kids and aging parents. It is not until some point in our fifties or sixties that most of us will start to notice a decrease in our energy level, and begin making necessary adjustments to deal with it.

Cancer treatment offers no such transition period. It forces you, in a very abrupt way, to face your depleted energy. All of a sudden, you notice you can't keep up. You feel out of sync with others your age—and with your old self. Friends and loved ones may not always understand this, and will say things like, "Oh, just get a little rest" or "How bad could it be?" Unless they've been there they have no frame of reference for how devastatingly cancer can impact your energy level, just like you didn't before starting treatment. They may think you're experiencing a "normal" tired feeling, not the overwhelming exhaustion of cancer-related fatigue.

Tips and Suggestions

Here are some ideas and general recommendations for dealing with cancer-related fatigue:

- Check for other possible medical factors. Let your medical team know when you are overly fatigued, especially if your CRF is much worse than during previous chemo cycles. Your team may want to look into any underlying medical reasons (e.g., if chemo is affecting your blood counts and you're anemic, or if you're experiencing thyroid function changes).

- Make sure to keep up your nutritional intake and drink plenty of fluids during chemo, because a lack of either can contribute to fatigue.

- Keep a diary—whether on your phone or tablet or in a paper journal—to track those times when your energy level is higher or lower during each chemotherapy cycle. Plan your most important tasks and activities for when your energy is at its peak—usually right before your next round of chemo begins.

- When approaching a day in your cycle when you are likely to feel totally exhausted, prioritize those basic activities that you *need* to take care of—like showering and eating—and leave more serious tasks for later.

- If you have something you really want to do on a particular evening, take it easy earlier in the day so you have enough reserve energy to draw on come nighttime.

- Contrary to what you may think, physical activity like walking can actually help with cancer-related fatigue. What's critically important is to listen to your body. There may be several days during each treatment cycle when you really just need to sleep and rest, and that's okay. Then, when you start feeling better, you can try incorporating more walking into your routine— within your home, going up and down stairs, or walking outside and around the block.

- If you're somebody who's used to exercising *a lot*, ask your oncology team what's appropriate during this period. Cancer centers have great resources to guide you, and some even have fitness classes specially designed for those in the midst of active treatment.

- In between treatments, write out or make a recording describing how great you feel after recovering from a really rough bout of fatigue. Then, the next time you're in the middle of a CRF episode during your chemo cycle, reading or listening to these affirmations will remind you that no matter how terrible you feel *now*, you're eventually going to get better—just like you did the last time.

- Create several playlists—one with mellow songs, one with more energetic and upbeat tunes, and another with background music—to listen to at different points in your treatment cycle, depending on your mood and fatigue level.
- Acupuncture and massage—under the care of acupuncturists and massage therapists specifically trained to work with oncology patients—can help with fatigue. I have patients who swear by weekly acupuncture and therapeutic massage during treatment. Just make sure these integrative therapies are done in conjunction with your oncology team by professionals who really understand your specific cancer.

Remember, there is no one right way to fight CRF. What works best for my patients is trying several different methods, at different times, and seeing which are most effective for them. You'll likely find that it is a combination of things.

Cognitive Changes (Chemo Brain)

It is common during treatment to find that you are foggier cognitively. This condition is officially known as cancer-related cognitive impairment (CRCI), but most people just call it "chemo brain" (though people undergoing radiation therapy and other treatments can also experience it).

The causes of chemo brain vary and are not well understood, and multiple factors may contribute. For example, when you're really anxious, it can be very hard to process information and focus on tasks. Similarly, one of the symptoms of depression can be difficulty focusing or concentrating. If you're fatigued or have trouble sleeping, you naturally have cognitive fatigue as well. If you're in pain of any sort—even a mild, dull pain that doesn't go away—it is going to affect your ability to home in on things and function at your best. Think about your past experiences; if you had a dull headache or a toothache, for instance, it was hard to concentrate on anything else. It's the same thing with cancer. Multiple variables can impact your ability to focus and pay attention so you can assimilate information.

Common Symptoms

How does chemo brain manifest? Your concentration and focus may be different. You may be unable to read for long periods, or find you don't remember something you just read—and have to go back and reread it several times. You may be watching TV but notice midway through a show that your concentration is shot and you can't follow along. I often tell people to try and avoid reading or watching anything during treatment that is particularly taxing and complicated. Very short articles or silly comedies are probably the best choice.

You may also experience memory and word-finding difficulties. Words will be "on the tip of your tongue" but you won't be able to remember them. In addition, while multitasking is something you may have once done with ease, you might now get easily confused when dealing with several things at once. If you try and plan ahead, you could become overwhelmed. It may feel, in computer terms, like your processing speed is slower. This can be especially frustrating because young adulthood is a time when the human brain naturally functions and processes information quickly. While chemo brain changes may be subtle, and others will tell you they don't notice them, you *do* notice them. That, in turn, impacts how you feel—and how you function.

Tips and Suggestions

As debilitating as it can be, chemo brain is usually temporary. Managing your stress can really help, so get treatment for your anxiety, depression, and pain. Fatigue can also interfere with your ability to function cognitively, so if there are certain cognitive tasks that you need to do, learn to pace yourself in terms of how you use your energy.

Here are a few tips that may help you cope with chemo brain:

- Write yourself reminder notes, even for routine tasks. This is usually not something that young adults, particularly those under thirty, are accustomed to doing, but give it a try.
- Put the reminders around your house—perhaps on sticky notes—where you can spot them easily.
- Repeat what you want to remember. Sometimes patients tell me about walking to another room to do something and forgetting what it is by the time they get there. Repeating what you're doing as you make this trip might help.
- Try some of the great phone and desktop apps designed to help you organize and review information.
- If apps seem too overwhelming at first, set up reminder alarms on your phone.
- Break down tasks into smaller, more manageable chunks. Number each step.

The reasons for CRCI during treatment may be different than *post*-treatment causes, which we will discuss in a later chapter.

Integrative Medicine

Known primarily until recent years as complementary therapy, integrative medicine can be used during or after cancer treatment—and includes a wide array of different approaches. In some cases, these are offered directly at your cancer center or an affiliated academic medical center; if not, your oncology team should be able to connect you with an outside integrative medicine practice.

Among the integrative medicine modalities (also known as integrative therapies) used in conjunction with cancer care are:

- **Acupuncture:** Research shows that acupuncture can help you with nausea, vomiting, sleep issues, anxiety, and pain related to cancer treatment. Many of my patients have acupuncture treatments in between their chemotherapy appointments, as part of their self-care routines, and they really feel that it helps reduce their nausea and improve their energy after chemo. Often they also feel calmer, more relaxed, and better overall.

- **Therapeutic massage:** A massage can be relaxing, but it can also help treat symptoms such as lymphedema or pain. As with a mental health professional, you want to make sure you see a massage therapist who understands the cancer treatment or surgery you are having and knows how to work with you.
- **Meditation, expressive arts, and exercise:** All of these approaches, which we discuss in other chapters, are extremely beneficial for many cancer patients. Hospitals may group these practices as part of integrative medicine along with acupuncture and massage.

Whichever integrative therapy or therapies you choose to explore, it is important that you see a practitioner who either works at a cancer center or academic medical center or is somebody your oncology team has trained or previously worked with. As with mental health professionals, some integrative therapy practitioners don't really understand cancer and cancer treatment. Then there are the "experts" who will make outrageous claims about herbs and supplements, recommendations that may actually do more harm than good. These individuals will think nothing of exploiting you during a very vulnerable time in your life for their own financial gain, so always make sure you have a strong reference before meeting with any outside practitioners.

You can find in the Resources section a variety of facilities offering comprehensive integrative medicine services specifically for cancer patients and their families. Remember, it doesn't matter if someone has an office close to your home, or is even willing to make house calls. What's important is that you get the safest and most clinically sound treatment, *not* the most convenient.

Understanding Targeted Therapies and Immunotherapies

I want to briefly touch on targeted therapies and immunotherapies. It is beyond the scope of this book to go into detail about these treatments, which are constantly evolving, but there is a possibility your oncologist may offer one or more of these if indicated.

Targeted Therapies

Also known as precision oncology, targeted therapies home in on specific molecules that cancer cells need to grow and spread. Initially, the medical establishment thought that targeted therapies would be less toxic than chemotherapies. Unfortunately, that is not the case. There is variability in terms of side effects, just as there can be with chemo, because different types of targeted therapies use different mechanisms of action. Some of the side effects are similar to those experienced with chemo, such as diarrhea, fatigue, and changes in blood counts.

Immunotherapies

Immunotherapies boost and use your body's own immune system to identify and attack cancer cells. They consist of a variety of treatments, including vaccines and CAR T-cell therapy. Again, while initially thought to be less toxic than chemo, immunotherapies are also associated with fatigue, nausea, diarrhea, achy muscles and joints, mouth sores, and skin reactions such as rashes.

Stem Cell Transplant

Your bone marrow produces your red and white blood cells and platelets. If your bone marrow becomes unhealthy due to a blood disorder or a cancer, such as leukemia, a bone marrow transplant (BMT)/stem cell transplant may be indicated. Your unhealthy marrow is replaced with healthy stem cells either from a donor (allogeneic) or your own (autologous). Undergoing a BMT is an arduous process, usually requiring several weeks of hospitalization to undergo high-dose chemotherapy and/or radiation followed by careful monitoring for about a year. Recovery is gradual and can be slow. Risks include infection and graft-versus-host disease (GVHD), a condition that can happen with allogeneic transplants in which the donor's cells attack the patient's body. Some GVHD is expected, but at times it can become problematic and longer lasting. Speaking with a psychologist or social worker pre-transplant to help you prepare, along with a consultation post-transplant, can assist you with the after-effects. Additional resources offered to you may include dietitians (GVHD can affect the GI system), sexual health (to deal with genital GVHD), PT, and OT. BMTInfonet.org is a good resource.

Remember that no matter which treatment, or combination of treatments, your cancer journey entails, you are not alone. There are many others dealing with similar challenges and people on your clinical team and in your life willing to help. In the chapters to come, we will explore how to handle the emotional and physical changes that arise during—and after—treatment, and how to care for yourself as you go through them.

Key Points

- The media and popular culture portray cancer treatment in terrifying and nerve-racking ways, and while treatment is certainly very difficult, there have been great advances made to help you manage and recover.
- Knowing what to expect in terms of potential side effects during different treatments can help you to anticipate possible challenges—and seek out ways to deal with them.
- Remember, side effects *will* get better. Understanding the typical time frames for side effects, and the recuperation necessary for each, can help, as will reminding yourself that as bad as you feel now, it won't last forever.
- Fatigue, might be a new feeling for you, and it can interfere greatly with your ability to live life on your terms.
- Whatever feelings you are experiencing are appropriate. There are no right or wrong emotions as you go through treatment.

CHAPTER 5
Emotional and Life Changes

Keisha, twenty-four, was referred to me right after learning she had acute myeloid leukemia (AML). She was nearing the completion of her master's degree in social work when diagnosed, and was upset about the major disruptions that AML treatment—which included a stem cell transplant—was causing her academically and emotionally.

We handled her issues at school by figuring out which classes Keisha could most easily drop if necessary and how she could seek accommodations (like extra time on projects) with her professors and school administrators. The bigger challenge, it turned out, was the difficulties she was having sharing her true feelings with those closest to her.

"My family is very supportive, but they don't like hearing me say anything about being scared," Keisha told me. "I'm hoping for a good outcome, but I'm also terrified about my long-term prognosis. Every time I try and express my fears, they just hush me up and say everything is going to be okay."

In our first several sessions, Keisha and I spent considerable time on "normalizing" her feelings. I assured her it was totally understandable to have such emotions, and we explored ways she could handle her family's overly upbeat attitude—including telling them it was more hurtful than helpful. When she shared how much she missed her friends while in recovery, and longed to talk to someone who really understood what she was going through, I connected her with our Young Adult Program and a support group focused on dealing with stem cell transplants. This all seemed to help her, as did moving in with her grandmother to be closer to treatment leading up to her transplant.

A little later on, her grandmother became concerned about how much Keisha—normally reserved and easygoing—was lashing out at her aggressively. Reviewing Keisha's medications, we realized she was on a high dose of steroids to ward off graft-versus-host disease after her transplant. Such a dosage can cause irritability, anger, restlessness, sleep disturbance, and mood changes.

"My grandmother and I came into the cancer center together and discussed with the oncology team ways to cope with the side effects while the team worked on adjusting my meds," recalls Keisha. "Openly talking and coming up with a plan felt much better than not sharing."

Acknowledging Your Emotions

Sometimes when a young adult who has just been diagnosed with cancer is sent to me, the conversation will start something like this:

"So, how are you feeling?"

"Fine."

"Really? That's surprising, since you just found out you have cancer."

I'm not trying to make light of the situation by responding this way. I'm hoping that, upon reflection, the individual I'm meeting with will realize that most people are *not* going to feel "fine" when told they have cancer—especially when that diagnosis shocks them in the prime of their lives. By bringing this out in the open, I'm letting them know that if they want to share whatever they are really going through emotionally, they are in a safe place to do so.

The fact is, there is no "right" way to feel. From your initial cancer workup throughout your treatment and beyond, it is normal to experience a wide range of emotions: fear, anger, sadness, disbelief, frustration—and more. All of them are valid. Don't ever be ashamed of them or let anybody judge you for having them. I sometimes find that young adult patients don't know what they feel or need because cancer can be so confusing. I often provide psychoeducation to help them understand what they are feeling, giving them a name and a framework to make sense of their emotions.

It's Okay Not to Share

Not everybody spends time going through their feelings and then wants to share them—with a psychologist or anybody else. That's okay too. Some of you, once you know your treatment plan, will just focus on getting through it. Cancer is viewed as an inconvenience to your life, something you need to endure, but you don't want to dwell or talk about it. You're going to continue going to work, or school, and will only share the details about your situation with those closest to you. If people ask how you feel, you'll say, "Thanks for your concern. I'm okay."

You may deal this way with your feelings because that's how you normally handle them. You're not someone who reflects on emotions much. Perhaps you have many life stressors already, and cancer is just one more thing on your list. You've got aging parents, other family members with medical issues, or financial problems, and you need to compartmentalize your cancer rather than focus on it. Maybe, because of your religious or spiritual views, you find "praying on it" is more comfortable, and helpful, than exploring your feelings by yourself or with someone else. Whatever approach you are taking, as long as it is working for you and not compromising your health or safety, that's fine. There is no reason to feel you *need to* reflect on what's happening by meeting with a therapist, a support group, or anybody else. Once your active cancer treatment is over, you may find you want to go back and process your emotions.

At this point I think sharing an experience from my own childhood might be helpful. My mother was diagnosed with head and neck cancer when she was twenty-six, and in the next two years went through two recurrences. At the time of the last recurrence, when I was four years old, the tumor was growing so fast that she needed to undergo a major surgery while pregnant with my younger brother. As if that was not stressful enough, a year before this my mother had lost her only sibling in an unexpected tragedy. So she had a young child (me), was pregnant, was dealing with a major loss, *and* was having a serious cancer surgery that would result in significant disability.

This was the late 1960s, when there was not a lot of focus on the emotional side of going through cancer. But that was not how my mom coped anyway. She had a very strong religious faith and during this period went on several church retreats with my father geared toward young adult couples. Maybe she shared her feelings with her priest, but at no point do I believe she ever discussed them with a medical professional. In fact, I don't remember her speaking to *anybody* about her cancer. Once she went through her last surgery and rehabilitation and was able to grow her hair long enough to cover the scar that ran all down her neck, she never mentioned cancer unless it was time for her yearly checkups—and then only to complain about the hassle of needing to take the time to go.

When, in her late seventies, my mom was diagnosed with a totally different cancer—breast cancer—she chose to deal with it in the same way. She never attended a support group, went to a breast cancer fundraiser, or wore a pink shirt or ribbon. Her focus was on getting through the treatment and getting on with her life.

Mom did not want the cancer to interfere with her daily routine any more than it had to, and she didn't want to talk about it other than to get treatment- and side effect–related information. When I asked her why, she told me, "I don't believe thinking and talking about my feelings is helpful. I just want to live my life." I'm not saying how my mother handled things was right or wrong, or the best way, but it was *her* way. It's important to accept—and respect—every individual's means of dealing as long as it does not impact their treatment or their caregivers in a negative way. Don't interfere, as long as it's working.

My mother's way of managing is certainly not unique. Take the patient who first came to see me after being diagnosed with a gynecological cancer the summer before starting college. This young woman had surgery that same summer and then needed the equivalent of a semester's worth of chemotherapy infusions. Rather than delay her freshman year, which would have been totally understandable, she started school and chemo at the same time—and didn't share her situation with anybody other than her advisor, her professors, and her roommate. Her treatment day was Friday, so her professors knew she'd be out that day each cycle. She got some extra time for papers and exams and, in the end, managed to go through the entire semester with almost nobody outside this small circle finding out.

This was in direct contrast to another of my patients, who also started college while going through cancer treatment. When she lost her hair during her first semester of freshman year, this woman chose not to wear a wig because she found it uncomfortable and didn't feel the need to hide her thinning hair. She explored with me what the experience of having cancer was doing to her life, how it was affecting her peer relationships, and how much it had changed her—at least temporarily—from the athletic, outgoing person she had been in high school. She felt a lot of anger about what was going on, and the two of us discussed that while these feelings were completely understandable, and appropriate, they could change over time. This is true for everyone. As we touched on before, you can expect all types of emotions at different points in your cancer trajectory, and it's important to acknowledge and accept these emotions for what they are—*your* thoughts and *your* feelings.

Practice Accepting Emotions

If the idea of dealing with your emotions doesn't come naturally, you're not alone. If you are interested, this exercise might help you start to become more comfortable with addressing them. When you feel a certain emotion coming on, rather than pushing it aside or letting it overwhelm you, just try to pull back, observe your emotion, and acknowledge/accept it. This doesn't mean you have to *like* it; rather, it means noticing and observing your emotion rather than "becoming the emotion" and being consumed by it.

Whether out loud or in your head, state to yourself exactly what's happening:

- "I'm having a feeling of fear right now."
- "I am noticing sadness right now."

- "I realize that at this moment, my thoughts are going round and round in my mind and I am experiencing lots of feelings."

In some cases, as in the third example, your specific feelings at any one moment may not be so easy to identify. As human beings we feel a wide range of emotions, and emotions can be very complicated. You may feel relieved about having completed two cycles of chemotherapy, but also frustrated because you still have four cycles to go. It's okay to have two opposite emotions at the same time. The world—and life—is not black-and-white. It's not always "or"; it can also be "and." You are not necessarily feeling happy or sad; you can be feeling happy *and* sad. There is no such thing as "good" or "bad" emotions. They are *your* emotions, and being able to accept them for what they are can be helpful in dealing with the ups and downs of treatment.

Toxic Positivity, or the Tyranny of Positive Thinking

Unfortunately, society *does* attach judgment to emotions, and that can make it very hard for you to experience what you're feeling. One way this judgment can arise is through toxic positivity.

What Is Toxic Positivity—and What Does It Sound Like?

Toxic positivity involves someone negating or suppressing the painful and often very appropriate emotions that come with a traumatic event, such as cancer, by insisting that the individual experiencing it focus on the positive. If you tell them you're upset about a bad scan, for example, they will offer some simple platitude like, "Don't worry—everything happens for a reason." It's like they are making a decree: Only positive vibes here!

Patients ask me all the time: "Are my feelings normal? Are they justified?" Yes, your feelings are justified. You don't need to prove them to others. You are human. When people challenge you through toxic positivity, it shuts down the conversation. It does not allow you to express the range of emotions you may have about your cancer, which are totally expected—especially at this time in your life, when cancer is totally *unexpected*. Toxic positivity rejects genuine concerns such as sadness and anger that we all feel when facing extremely difficult situations.

Whether they realize it or not, those practicing toxic positivity are asking you to ignore, negate, and suppress your emotions by saying things like:

- "Be glad you got the *good* cancer. The survivorship rate is much better."
- "You're so lucky! You didn't lose all your hair from chemo."
- "Don't worry, this experience will make you stronger."

As a cancer patient, statements like these—however well intentioned—can make you feel isolated and alone. You're expressing anger, or fear, or sadness, and this individual is not validating you. It's a form of gaslighting, in that the other person is trying to manipulate you into believing your response and emotions are wrong. You may think, "*Am* I overreacting? Maybe I *do* have the 'good cancer.'" Sure, maybe you did not lose your hair, but that doesn't mean everything is okay. Whether or not they realize it, or will admit to it, people practicing toxic positivity are dismissing your feelings and experiences by making *you* question them.

Comments like, "Everything happens for a reason" or "It's all going to be okay" can be frustrating or even infuriating. I mean, what possible reason *could* there be for this to happen to you? How do *they* know it's all going to be okay? Can they predict the future? It's completely understandable to be annoyed by such platitudes.

Why Do People Express Toxic Positivity?

There are many reasons people might say these things. Certainly most of them believe they are being helpful. If it's a younger person, I think it's partly because they likely have no emotional reference point in terms of what you're going through. They just don't *get it*. They have no way to truly feel what it's like to have cancer at your age, since they have not experienced anything similar. Because they are so uncomfortable and don't know what to say, they'll express some sort of empty platitude rather than say nothing.

Another possibility is that they could be the type who doesn't really reflect that much on their own range of human emotions, and are just trying to keep things positive while talking to you. Those who are religious may think it's comforting to say, "God never gives you more than you can handle." But even if you are religious, and have a strong sense of faith, you can *still* feel sad or angry that this burden has been thrust upon you. What has worked for them may not work for you in the same way.

There may be people in your life who have a particularly hard time hearing you express the emotions that come along with a cancer diagnosis. I see this often in parents of young adults. They hear their child say, "I'm so terrified" or "I don't want to die," and they don't know how to respond. It's so painful to see their child suffering, they will just say something like, "Don't worry. It's going to be okay."

If you've experienced this, it's understandable to feel hurt by it—but it is also important to remember that such reactions may be coming from a good place. People in your life, especially those closest to you, can have a very hard time dealing and coping with what's happening. So as your parents (or your sibling, or your best friend, or your partner), they are likely saying such things not only to try and comfort you, but also to comfort *themselves*. They are struggling with seeing and hearing you crying, or scared, and don't even want to consider you not being in their lives. They feel compelled to shut down the conversation and wipe those thoughts from their minds, and hope that an empty comment will provide that type of self-preservation. I am not making an excuse for how they are acting, but rather providing a possible explanation.

Patient Voices

"They do not ask me how I am,
but they tell me how to feel.
They do not want to know that I am weak,
so they tell me I am strong.
They do not want to know that I am scared,
so they tell me I am brave.
They do not want to know I am losing hope,
so they tell me I am inspiring.
They do not ask how I am,
because they cannot grasp how I am."
—Madison C.

Replying to Toxic Positivity

How you might respond to toxic positivity depends on the situation. You may not have the strength to educate and explain to people how their comments make you feel. In those cases, it's fine to just stay quiet, not say anything, and leave it at that. If you would like to try to improve things in the long term, however, you could offer some suggestions. One way I work to help family and friends of patients become more supportive toward their loved one dealing with cancer is by providing a crash course in communication skills. While each individual and situation is unique, there are certain statements and actions that I've found to be especially effective across the board when talking with people who might be struggling. Others are definite no-nos.

Examples of Unhelpful Emotional Support

You might want to consider passing along these as examples of what *not* to say:

- Useless platitudes like: "It's going to get better." (How do they know?) "I know just how you feel." (They do not—unless they've had the same cancer at the same age.) "Everything happens for a reason." (Oh, yeah? Prove it.)

- Offering unsolicited advice—if you don't ask for it, they shouldn't give it.
- Using words like "brave" and "strong" to describe your resiliency; these have become so overused they often make patients cringe.
- Suppressing or avoiding all negative emotions and encouraging you to "look on the bright side."
- Sharing stories of other people they know with cancer who had complications or died. You'd be amazed how often this happens, because a person's gut instinct on the spot may be to find a story to connect to your situation—without thinking through how that story ended until it's too late.

It is only natural for someone to want to say or do whatever they can to make you feel better, but these well-intentioned words don't usually work.

Examples of Helpful Emotional Support

Your loved ones might also appreciate hearing what kinds of words *are* helpful to you. These conversations can be a little awkward, but in the long run, everyone will likely benefit. Here are some things you could say if someone close to you engages in toxic positivity:

- Suggest that rather than asking, "How can I help?" they might try coming up with a list of ways they *can* help, and letting you decide. Even at the end of treatment, people need plenty of support—but the further they get away from treatment, the less often people check in on them.
- If they notice you are having a bad day, they could say, "Know that I am here for you."
- Tell them, "I know you are trying to make me feel better, but those words don't help. Are you able to just let me share my feelings?"
- Or say, "Can you just listen? That would be most helpful."
- Or maybe, "I don't need you to try and fix how I am feeling. Can you just sit with me and hold my hand?"

- Recommend that they listen and be silent if they're not sure what to say. Just being present is enough for someone going through a tough time. It's about the human connection. Ask if they can try to resist their desire to try to fix the situation, which is often unfixable.

People who love you and are struggling themselves with your cancer treatment may very well appreciate your being honest like this. By explaining how you feel, you might help them see the tremendous benefits of thinking before they speak. It's certainly worth a try.

If it is somebody you are *not* close to who is offering up the empty comments, you might want to use a different approach. Try one of these responses:

- "I know it's hard to see what I'm going through, and you may not know quite what to say. I would really appreciate if you could just listen."
- "It's hard to always look at the bright side when I have no hair, feel sick a lot of the time, and am missing out on my life. I know you are trying to be helpful, but perhaps think about how *you* would feel in my situation."
- "Yes, I understand it *could* be worse, but what I am going through is still challenging."

These are just suggestions; there is no correct or wrong way to respond. And as stated earlier, if it seems like an additional burden to try and share or teach people the best way to act around you, feel free to *not* respond and just let it go for the time being. You can always revisit things later, when you have more energy or interest.

Cancer the Interrupter—and Disrupter

As you deal with the emotional challenges of going through cancer, you're also facing a drastic upheaval of your life in general. Prior to your diagnosis, you may have been enjoying a series of predictable and enjoyable routines. Now cancer has suddenly come along and created chaos. Your full calendar is being disrupted by infusions, checkups, and other appointments, and you're finding yourself forced to constantly put things on hold. Whether it's your social life (relationships with peers, dating, travel), your practical life (school, work, finances), your emotional life (self-esteem, body image, sense of identity), or your ability to deal with treatment itself and all of its side effects, it feels like cancer is taking over every aspect of your existence. If you have preexisting medical issues, or have previously dealt with anxiety, depression, or substance abuse, these conditions can reemerge or be exacerbated as well. And because these different realms of your life overlap and affect one another regularly, the disruptions caused by cancer often become magnified.

It can all feel very overwhelming—and unfair. That's why learning how to balance your "cancer life" with your "normal life"—and integrating the two as best as possible—is critically important to getting through this challenging time. Rather than shutting your world down completely during treatment, explore different adjustments you can make so that you can continue doing what's most important. While it might be tough to ask for assistance, and not something you're accustomed to, you may be surprised by how people are willing to help you in this pursuit.

Here are some examples:

- **If you're in school,** notify the administration of your need for accommodations, seek out extensions on assignments or time accommodations for tests from your professors, perhaps drop a class, or even consider taking a semester off. You should be able to get tuition reimbursement or deferrals for serious medical issues (check with your school's bursar's office). Your treatment team can provide a letter or other documentation as needed. Many colleges, universities, and trade schools offer virtual classes, so that's another option to explore.

- **If you're working,** consider shifting to a part-time schedule for a period, or getting your chemotherapy infusions close to weekends to minimize the number of sick or half days you need off. If you find it necessary to take a long period of full days off, you could be eligible for up to twelve weeks of unpaid, job-protected leave under the federal Family and Medical Leave Act (FMLA). The FMLA only applies to private companies of fifty or more employees, but several states have extended this benefit to *all* private employees. In some cases, paid medical leave may also be available (check with your employer). Consider applying for short- or long-term disability and explore your other options.

- **If you're planning a big trip,** check in with your clinical team before assuming you need to cancel it. If your trip is planned around a special event, like a family wedding, your team may be able to adjust your chemotherapy cycle or other treatment so that you can attend and feel at your best (the more advanced notice you can give them, the better). If your team indicates that long trips are not advisable for a certain period, plan a series of smaller weekend or day outings.

- **If you enjoy exercising,** find ways to alter your workouts during treatment. If you're used to running marathons, train for a 3K or walk three times a week instead. If you normally go to the gym four days per week, shoot for one or two. Many cancer centers have exercise classes designed specifically for patients, led by experts who can help find the best fit for you depending on your type of cancer and treatment schedule.

Facing Changes in Your Autonomy

One of the biggest disruptions caused by cancer is what it does to your autonomy. Young adulthood is a period when you are naturally becoming more and more independent. In your twenties, you're often establishing yourself as separate from your parents or family of origin. In your thirties and forties, you may have a partner, kids, and/or colleagues who need and depend on you. You are probably accustomed to being in situations where you have the ability to make your own decisions, both about what you're doing now and what you *want* to do down the road. Now this unexpected interruption is interfering with those plans as well as your everyday life.

Whether you're eighteen, forty-nine, or anywhere in between when diagnosed, it is likely that cancer will at least temporarily derail a major developmental milestone—and the independence that comes with it. Instead of doing things on your terms and timetable, you're suddenly thrust into the position of asking others for support and ceding some of your autonomy.

Parents As Roommates

If you live on your own, your parents might suggest—or strongly encourage—that you move back in with them during treatment. This is a very common reaction. While getting rides to the cancer center, free laundry, and home-cooked meals is great, this could feel like a return to old family dynamics and a sense that you're regressing into a role you thought you'd left behind forever. Your parents will often insist on coming with you to medical appointments and try to take the lead in discussions with your clinical team as if you were all back in the pediatrician's office during grade school.

If you have your own home and/or family, a parent or sibling might move in with you to help out instead. This may not seem as challenging a scenario as you moving home, but believe me when I say that you will *always* be your parent's child. I've had forty-five-year-old patients tell me they felt infantilized by well-meaning moms and dads during cancer treatment. In some families, it's easier to maintain age-appropriate boundaries than others, and just like in any relationship, you may want to consider when and where to pick your battles. So should your spouse or partner, who, while no doubt appreciative of the help your family is providing, will likely butt heads with them sometimes around what's "best" for you during treatment.

Here are some ideas that might help you in meeting these challenges:

- Have a close friend—or "family of friends"—step in as your temporary roommate instead of a parent or sibling, thus alleviating the potential for old childhood dynamics to resurface.
- Try switching off between your parents (or siblings) caring for you, so there is less likely to be an opportunity for regressing into old familial roles.
- If you do move in with friends/family during your treatment and recovery, set up shared and private spaces so that you know you always have somewhere to go and be alone if needed.
- Before dramatically changing any living arrangements, try devising a schedule when parents/siblings/friends can come by to help you at crucial points of the day or week. You might find such visits are enough.

The key in all these scenarios is finding ways to set boundaries. While your cancer treatment, by its very nature, will include times when you are required to be cared for, that doesn't mean you have to completely lose your independence. Like most things in life, autonomy is not an "all-or-none" condition. Think of it as being on a continuum, and search for that place where both you and those who care about you can feel comfortable—and where your health and safety are assured.

Support (and Supporters) Comes in Different Forms

These situations are complicated: You may feel like a burden. Those who love you want to help, but you might not be used to this type of support since becoming an adult. It's important to remember that those close to you are scared about what's happening, just like you are, and are unsure of what to do. They wish they could just get rid of the cancer altogether for you. I've heard parents say, "It should be happening to *me*, not to my child." Since they can't make that happen, your family—and friends—want to do the next best thing, whatever that is.

In times like these, try and find ways to help your loved ones feel useful. Different people can do different things. Remember in Chapter 3 when we talked about having one person help write your "I've been diagnosed with cancer" emails, and another provide ongoing updates? It's the same situation here. There are numerous ways that people can assist you during treatment, some of which come easier than others depending on the individual. Organizations, whether cancer based or not, can also be a great means of social support.

Try to think of support as being divided up into three main areas:

- **Instrumental support** comes in the form of very tangible, functional tasks. Driving you to appointments. Bringing you food. Doing your shopping or laundry. Giving you financial assistance for help with rent or car payments or groceries.
- **Emotional support** is more about feelings than tasks. Listening to you. Letting you share your hopes and fears. Providing you with a sense of security. Holding you as you cry.
- **Informational support** is what someone can offer you in the way of resources. Links to support groups. Connections to a great doctor, physical therapist, or acupuncturist. Insurance or financial advice.

While there may be some people who can truly provide all three, most friends and family will likely be more comfortable—and successful—helping you in one specific way. Not everyone is "good" at emotional support or has the financial resources to pay your electric bill. Do your best when possible to match people up according to the type of help that is easiest for them to provide.

Navigating Difficult Family Situations

All families are complicated. There may be certain individuals, including members of your close family, who are incapable of giving support in a way that is helpful to you. In some cases, even if they try, it only winds up hurting more than helping. A major part of my therapy sessions with young adults is focused on managing and coping with family dynamics during cancer treatment. In times of major stress like this, it's hard to know how best to involve, or not involve, particular family members.

My advice is that, when possible, try first to establish boundaries that allow challenging family members to feel they are offering healthy support—but with some emotional and/or physical distance. If this approach becomes untenable, and is causing you too much distress, you may need to minimize or discontinue your interactions with these individuals—perhaps just for the time being—for your own welfare. Keep this in mind: If there is one time in your life when you need to do what is best *for you*, it is during cancer treatment.

At times it is not just one or two family members, but most of your family, that is problematic. That's when it is important to remember something else: Sometimes it's the family you *choose*, rather than the one you were born into, that is really there for you.

Social Media and the Fear of Missing Out (FOMO)

Dealing with cancer is now likely consuming a large part of your time and energy. Even if the rest of your life isn't completely on hold, it has likely changed significantly. Of course, many people these days chronicle their lives on social media, but posting updates might be difficult for you now. In addition, seeing others posting about their "normal" lives can be upsetting.

It is important to keep in mind, however, that all is not necessarily as it seems. A social media post is not representative of all that is really happening to a person at a given moment, and should not interfere with how you look at your own life either. The woman smiling on Instagram or Facebook as she dines with friends in a trendy new restaurant could also be dealing with a sick parent. There is no way of knowing how happy a poster *really* is, or all that's going on in their lives.

The natural reaction when you see upbeat posts, of course, is to wish you were doing those fun things too. This fear of missing out, or FOMO, is a universal experience, but you may find it happening more often as a cancer patient. Seeing your peers enjoying themselves out on the town, on vacation, and marking occasions like graduations, weddings, new jobs, and new babies while you watch on from an infusion chair or hospital bed can make you feel like everybody is moving forward while you're stuck in place.

Cancer has forced you to pause your life, and it's only natural to feel pain and discomfort as you grapple with being out of sync. There is no way to completely avoid these emotions in the social media world, but here are some suggestions for dealing with them:

- Remind yourself that what people depict on social media are curated snapshots.
- Limit yourself to a specific amount of social media time each day. If you still feel a strong sense of FOMO, consider stopping altogether (at least temporarily).
- If you are comfortable sharing, and think it will help you feel better, create your own social media posts detailing your cancer journey in photos and narrative. Along with being healing, this approach can validate to others why you've had to temporarily pause your life.
- Explore alternative ways to stay connected with peers, like phone calls, Zoom calls, letters, and (when possible) in-person visits.

As we discussed earlier in this chapter regarding emotions in general, it's important to remember that all your feelings about social media—disappointment, anger, frustration, genuine happiness for someone's success—are valid. Rather than suppress them, try to acknowledge any emotions that arise. If you think it would help, talk through your feelings with others who may understand, such as fellow young adults with cancer.

Social Isolation

In general, feeling supported and having relationships with others has been shown to be an important component of living a healthy life. It is also beneficial for our *mental health*. Almost every time I talk to a young adult cancer patient, and in study after study conducted around this age group, the issue of isolation from peers comes up. This makes sense, because people ages eighteen to forty-nine are constantly developing and building social relationships—and a sense of connectedness. As you form your own identity and exert your independence, your circle widens beyond your parents and siblings to include friends, colleagues, partners, and perhaps children.

These relationships, in many cases, are formed by your emerging interests. If you're drawn to a particular sport, type of music, or hobby, you may form friendships and/or join groups centered around those activities. Fraternities, sororities, and clubs can provide a sense of togetherness in college, as can professional organizations offering camaraderie and networking opportunities in the working world. Similar-aged peers become your most important support system as you continue growing and experiencing new milestones.

Cancer's Impact on Your Social Life

Once cancer enters into your young adult life, it interrupts, disrupts, and delays this very natural part of your social-emotional development. While you may feel great support from your family and your oncology team as you go through treatment, you can at the same time experience a sense of isolation from your peers. You're no longer in sync with them, and they may not have the time or understanding needed to connect with you as you navigate your new circumstances. They might be coping with finals, collaborating on a big project at work, or getting their kid into pre-school, while you're navigating surgery, chemotherapy, or four straight weeks of radiation. You might even have to move away, either back in with your family and/or to be closer to your treatment center. No matter how far the physical distance, it can feel like a gulf is forming between you.

Studies have shown that for young adults with cancer, isolation from peers can have a major impact on their quality of life. When social isolation like this happened on a grand scale worldwide during the COVID-19 pandemic, young adults in particular suffered from being separated from one another. In that case, however, they were all going through roughly the same experience. Cancer is different.

Unless your friends are dealing with treatment themselves, it's nearly impossible for them to imagine what it's all about.

Patient Voices

"When weathering the ever-changing emotional storm that accompanies cancer, it can be tempting to withdraw—to self-isolate—since it seems like no one could understand your unique experience. But seeking out connection, whether with loved ones or within the YA cancer community, is the ultimate antidote to loneliness. Once I started getting really vulnerable with those closest to me, I could start moving past some of the fear and depression to re-access the joy in my life." —Colleen M.

Staying In Touch with Friends

I often explore with my patients what they can do to reduce these feelings of isolation. Here are a few suggestions:

- Even if you can't engage in the same number of activities as before due to your treatment schedule and/or lack of energy, try your best to stay involved with peers. If you are an officer in a club, for example, consider stepping back from that role but continuing to attend at least half the meetings. Or if you can't play pickleball with your friends, join them for lunch after the game when you're up to it.
- If you're just too tired to go *anywhere* in person, try and stay on the radar of different clubs and organizations through group emails, texts, or social media. If virtual attendance is an option, try that.
- Consider blogging or making videos to keep folks abreast of your life.

Exploring Young Adult Cancer Support Groups

Another way to avoid isolation is to join one of the many young adult cancer programs, which usually offer both traditional support groups as well as social and psycho-educational events. Many offer virtual gatherings, but it's great to attend in person if possible.

The key benefit of such groups and programs is that they provide the opportunity to connect with peers who are going through the same experiences and can understand and relate on a deep emotional level with what's happening to you. Even if they have a different type of cancer and/or treatment plan, there is a bond that comes with knowing they have endured a similar challenge during this transformative period in their lives. As I've seen many times with my own patients, being able to form these special relationships can be quite powerful and validating. These groups can take many shapes—from movie and art nights to book clubs and trivia challenges—and might be offered online, in person, or a hybrid.

While they may be focused more on engagement than entertainment, support groups can also be a great way to connect with people. These tend to be more young adult specific and usually have a clinician like myself serving as facilitator. Some meet for a set period (biweekly for eight sessions, for instance), while others are offered on an ongoing basis—with new people dropping in and out all the time. Seek out groups in which you'll both get something out of what other participants share and feel comfortable sharing yourself at some point, and don't worry if your first foray is not successful. Every group is different, and there are plenty of options out there. If you need help finding the right fit, ask your social worker or someone else on your clinical team. And check out the list of groups in the Resources section at the end of this book.

Financial Toxicity

We've covered in this chapter a wide array of ways that cancer touches your life, from the emotional roller coaster of diagnosis and treatment to changes in your independence level. Here's another: the impact on your finances. Cancer and its associated costs can lead to financial hardships and psychological distress for you, your family, and other caregivers. As with other topics, however, knowing what to expect and the resources available to you can go a long way toward minimizing the damage.

The Cost of Cancer

Cancer treatment–associated financial toxicity comes in two main forms:

- **Direct costs:** insurance, co-pays, medicines, home care, travel expenses, medical bills
- **Indirect costs:** lost work time (and income), missing out on promotions at work or interviews for new jobs, missing out on classes and activities at school, depleted savings

Financial toxicity is one of the most emotionally draining and stressful aspects of cancer care for young adults. It can greatly impact your quality of life, especially because this is a time when you might already be dealing with significant expenses and debt—from school loans to car payments to rent/mortgage, childcare, and weekly grocery bills. Even if you want to get a new job, or *second* job, to help deal with these challenges, the demands of your treatment often make it impossible to seek one out.

Although it can be a detriment to cancer patients of any age, financial toxicity tends to be more of a strain for those who are under fifty when diagnosed. Older adults have often paid down or eliminated some of life's larger expenditures and, in many cases, have become empty nesters with smaller homes and fewer mouths to feed. They also may have accumulated more savings to help them through if they need to take unpaid leave or travel for treatment. Younger adults, in contrast, may have no choice but to ask their parents for financial support or their old bedroom if they find themselves drowning under the costly demands of cancer care.

Finding Resources

Until recently, financial toxicity had not garnered much attention as a serious issue for cancer patients. Thankfully, this is no longer the case, and it is now being addressed as a part of supportive care by many cancer centers. One of the first things I do with new patients these days is introduce them to a resource specialist who can in turn connect them with outlets and programs designed to assist people facing financial hardships due to cancer. You can ask your care team if these specialists exist at your treatment center. At some centers, it may be a social worker who handles this role, and if you're not physically and/or emotionally up to meeting with them, they can consult with a member of your family or a friend.

There are also organizations and resources available. Whether it's through the American Cancer Society, the Leukemia and Lymphoma Society, or any of the many other private and nonprofit foundations set up to aid young adult cancer patients, there is help for everything from groceries to gasoline to affordable housing. In some cases, resource specialists or social workers can also help you look into temporary or long-term disability, connect you with a financial counselor, or provide insurance education. If you need to travel for your treatment, there is often free or discounted lodging available near many cancer centers as well.

Assistance can vary by type of cancer and state, so be sure to check if you meet the necessary requirements. (For a list of agencies set up to help patients, see the Resources section.)

Living with Uncertainty

Perhaps one of the most significant changes to your life when dealing with cancer is that you are now immersed in a world of uncertainty. Young adulthood is usually not a time in life when you give such emotions much thought. You're so engaged in doing, accomplishing, learning, and exploring that you can't imagine anything stopping you. In many countries, including the United States, society places a big emphasis on looking good, keeping active, and being vital. Consequently, in your twenties and thirties, mortality is primarily an abstract concept. Maybe if you're in your forties, with aging parents, you have been forced to think about it a bit more, but you're still not necessarily considering *your own* mortality. You're young, so it's only natural to think that you're in complete control of your destiny. You have certainty and can make choices.

Cancer, of course, changes all that. Death is no longer just an abstract concept, something you discuss in philosophy class, read about in a novel, or watch portrayed in a movie or play. Whereas you previously could not imagine in anything but a fleeting, abstract way the idea of leaving your loved ones alone, this thought is now suddenly and often very deeply imprinted on your mind—no matter your current prognosis. You've been forced by cancer to face the reality of your own mortality at a time when you're not really equipped to deal with it.

Now it feels like cancer has thrust these thoughts, and this awareness of life's frailty, to the forefront of your mind. Your peers are so focused on action and accomplishment that they don't have time to reflect on things in quite this way, which often leads to your feeling isolated from them.

While living with uncertainty is definitely difficult, and stressful, there are strategies you can use to manage your anxiety, practice self-care, and find ways (big and small) to engage with the world around you. By employing these techniques, which we will explore in the next chapter, you can bring joy and meaning to your life during this challenging time.

Key Points

- There is no "right" way to deal with your emotions—but it can help to accept them. Recognizing your feelings and acknowledging them to yourself is the first step in dealing with any fears and anxiety you may have around them.
- Don't let toxic positivity get you down. However well intentioned, overly optimistic platitudes from friends and family, like, "This experience will make you stronger" or "You got the *good* cancer," can make you feel hurt and misunderstood. When processing such comments—known as toxic

positivity—remember that nobody but you understands your true feelings.

- However awkward, try to call out toxic positivity when you can—and then provide tips to the perpetrators on more constructive communication methods and questions they could use in the future. Sometimes just quietly being there for (and with) you is best.
- Be open to help—but maintain your autonomy. There will often be times when you need support from others during your cancer trajectory, but it is important to set boundaries and retain your independence.
- Seek balance with your "cancer" and "normal" lives. A cancer diagnosis and treatment can cause chaos at school, at work, and in your social life, and the best way to deal with such disruptions is to try to meet them head-on when appropriate. It's often better to seek solutions than accept limitations.

CHAPTER 6
Well-Being, Mental Health, and Self-Care

As the oldest of four siblings with two working parents, Molly learned to care for others at an early age. She was the person everyone counted on and called, knowing she would be there for them, and this continued long into adulthood.

Molly was diagnosed with colon cancer at age forty-three, and I met her shortly thereafter. She told me she had been so consumed with raising two school-aged kids, working as an office manager at an insurance firm, and caring for her husband and extended family that she had ignored her changing bowel habits. Then, when blood began appearing in her stool, she assumed it was hemorrhoids (which she'd had delivering her children) and initially ignored this warning sign for cancer.

I asked what she did to relax and care for herself, and she just laughed. Along with everything else, she had a son on the autism spectrum who needed special attention at school and home, as well as older parents who had both recently undergone surgery.

"Even before my cancer diagnosis, I felt emotionally overloaded," recalls Molly. "So as I got near the end of chemotherapy, I wanted to see if I could start prioritizing those things that were most important to me and learn to better manage my stress."

The two of us went over Molly's lifestyle. She had trouble falling asleep because she worried a lot right before bed, and while she used to exercise regularly, she had gradually stopped doing so. We discussed possible self-care and stress-management behaviors she could incorporate into her daily routine, and decided on nightly diaphragmatic breathing (or belly breathing) and one yoga class a week.

"The belly breathing only took two or three minutes, which was the length of one song that I could listen to right before going to bed," recalls Molly. "Doing it then helped calm my mind and body to the point where I found it much easier to fall asleep."

On my suggestion, Molly found a friend to join her at the weekly yoga class. This turned out to be a strong motivator, and Molly noticed an uptick in her energy after just a few sessions. We also problem-solved around asking others to share some of the family-caregiver load. It took a while, but identifying her feelings and setting boundaries improved her emotional well-being—and got great results.

"My siblings agreed to take our parents to some of their medical appointments and help with their shopping, and I got my kids to do more chores around the house," Molly explains. "With additional time for myself, I got back to things I had missed for a long time, like playing cards with friends and attending church. I realized I could still be a good daughter, mom, wife, and sister without pushing myself to be superwoman."

Defining Mental Health and Self-Care

We've all heard the term "mental health," and the importance of practicing "self-care" is a hot topic nowadays. But do you know what these expressions actually mean? According to the National Institute of Mental Health (NIMH), "Mental health includes emotional, psychological, and social well-being. It is more than the absence of a mental illness—it's essential to your overall health and quality of life. Self-care can play a role in maintaining your mental health and help support your treatment and recovery if you have a mental illness." (I might add that self-care can also help you in dealing with a *physical* illness, such as cancer, that may be impacting your mental health and/or well-being.)

So what, exactly, is self-care? As defined by the NIMH, "Self-care means taking the time to do things that help you live well and improve both your physical health and mental health. This can help you manage stress, lower your risk of illness, and increase your energy. Even small acts of self-care in your daily life can have a big impact." Like Molly and most other young adults, you may be used to a harried lifestyle that doesn't provide time for self-care. After a cancer diagnosis, however, it is paramount that you *make* time, for the sake of yourself and those you care about. This chapter will focus on your overall health and well-being, with an emphasis on your mental health. It will help you examine the physical, emotional, psychological, social, and spiritual aspects of your life, and offer ways to incorporate self-care and stress management into your daily existence. After all, you can't really separate your physical health from your mental health. Together, they make up who you are as a human being.

Recognizing Your Emotions

You likely have myriad emotions swirling around at any given moment during your cancer journey—all of which can affect your mental health. In fact, sometimes you're experiencing so many different emotions—stress, fear, anger, concern—that it might feel impossible to keep track of them all. Then there are the additional "regular life" emotions that naturally arise. What if, in the middle of treatment, your partner suddenly tells you they can't cope with the situation, and ends your relationship? What if your best friend is getting married, but the wedding is scheduled for two days after your next chemotherapy treatment? Should you try and reschedule chemo, or just Zoom into the ceremony? How can you even begin to deal with all of these feelings?

Simply recognizing exactly what you feel, and why, might seem like a basic exercise, but it's not something that most of us really spend much time thinking about. Part of how you deal with your emotions is also what—or *who*—you attribute them to. Let's say you look at someone you find very attractive; your heart might start racing and your palms sweating because you're excited. On the other hand, you could also experience a racing heart and sweaty palms out of fear when facing somebody who is glaring menacingly at you. So, how you look at a situation, and how you interpret and attribute how you *feel*, influences both your emotions and your ability to process and deal with them.

You may often find yourself making such attributions quickly, and at times misattribute or misunderstand your feelings. For instance, while you might realize your increased heart rate comes from being scared, it may *also* be because you're excited—or it could be both. Taking a moment to become aware of precisely *what* you're feeling—and *why*—is a helpful first step in caring for your mental health.

Focus on What You Can Control

During young adulthood, you tend to think that you're totally in control, capable of making whatever choices you want. A cancer diagnosis, however, changes all that. You may suddenly experience an overwhelming feeling that what you've always believed is in fact an illusion. Ultimately, in terms of life and death, you are *not* in control. And while you likely already knew this intellectually, you suddenly understand it on a very real and experiential level.

Perhaps in the past you had a friend die by drowning, or in a car accident. In those fleeting moments, you might have felt this sense of powerlessness. Usually, however, such examples of life's precariousness are not a regular part of young adulthood.

Now it's different. Now you may be pondering profound and existential questions—as they relate to your *own* life and your *own* mortality. Such an awareness of control—or *lack* of control—can be very frightening. It may become all you think about, until you are so consumed and immobilized by this fear that you start missing out on life's day-to-day pleasures.

While it's normal during treatment to have emotions, stress, and fears, if you don't learn ways to cope with them, you may find yourself in a constant state of fight-or-flight—always looking for or expecting the next shoe to drop. The key to dealing with this level of stress is acknowledging that while you may not ultimately be in control of *all* aspects of your life with cancer, figuring out what you can't and can control can be extremely beneficial to living a healthy existence.

Stress and Cancer

When people start trying to figure this all out, finding a reason for why they got cancer may be a priority. A common question I get from patients is: "Did stress cause my cancer?" This requires a several-part answer.

"No, stress did not cause your cancer," I tell them. "But it's a complicated question."

Can Stress Cause Cancer?

There is no definitive evidence that stress directly causes cancer. Some research suggests stress can result in a suppression of the immune system. For instance, laboratory research has indicated that when investigators temporarily induce stress in rats, those rats' immune systems struggle and they seem to develop cancer at a higher rate. It is faulty logic, however, to make the leap from these studies to the conclusion that stress causes cancer in *humans*. First of all, we are not lab rats. Our emotions and our ways of responding to stress are much more complicated than those of rats. Second, other factors (not simply stress) can impact our immune systems. These include some health conditions such as diabetes and autoimmune illnesses, as well as environmental pollution, toxins, and vaccines. Third, this way of thinking does not take into account genetic variables associated with cancer. A temporary suppression of the immune system is but one factor in our complicated lives as human beings and the multitude of influences on our immune systems and bodies. So if there *is* any connection between stress and cancer, it is not a direct one.

Why, then, do people who hear this believe it? A big reason, I think, is because they want an explanation for why they have cancer. It goes back to control. If something has *caused* your cancer, then you can try to control it. Finding an explanation gives you a sense of agency over this and any related health problems. Much research, money, and energy has gone into examining this possible link, with plenty of articles and books presenting theoretical explanations for a direct link. Still, there has been no conclusive evidence one exists.

Stress Can Impact Your Health

Now here's the complicated part. While it's obvious that certain events like ending a relationship, losing a job, or dealing with financial instability can be stressful, so can "positive" things such as going away for college, starting an exciting new job, or having a baby. Stress is part of all our lives, and learning ways to cope with it can affect your health.

So while stress does not *cause* cancer, it can influence the cancer trajectory. In other words, how you perceive and address stress can have a ripple effect on your life that could lead to a cancer diagnosis—or, in some cases, a *later* cancer diagnosis.

Here's an example: A woman in her mid-forties came to see me after being diagnosed with stage III breast cancer. As she explained it, she had gotten so busy caring for her aging mother with Alzheimer's and her school-aged kids that she had skipped getting her annual mammograms for a couple of years. Stressed and emotionally overwhelmed with everything going on in her life, she did not make herself a priority. By the time she got around to having a mammogram, her cancer was at a more advanced stage than it likely would have been had she had an earlier screening.

I have also encountered individuals who developed cancer after engaging in risky behaviors for long periods of time. For example, if you deal with stress through heavy drinking, smoking, or taking serious drugs, there is a higher chance you could be diagnosed with cancer or another major health complication.

Addressing Stress During Treatment

How you handle stress *during* cancer treatment is another issue. You will almost certainly experience anxiety throughout this period, but if that stress reaches a point where you *avoid* your treatment—or don't adhere to it as prescribed—that, of course, will impact its effectiveness. It's the same issue if you don't take care of yourself as you go through cancer, or you continue to use drugs or drink alcohol heavily. Experiencing stress and difficult life situations is part of the "normal" human experience, but it is how you cope and behave in these circumstances that could impact how you respond to treatment.

Finding healthy ways to deal with the various stressors can help you during your recovery from cancer treatment—and beyond. The key is finding ways to manage your emotions even when feeling overwhelmed. When newly diagnosed patients tell me they feel out of control and uncertain about their lives, I suggest they try to acknowledge and examine those feelings. By learning to cope with your emotions, and *understand* them, you can discover how best to approach each new challenge cancer throws you.

When faced with a stressful and difficult situation, there are multiple ways to deal with it. One framework you might find helpful in figuring out how to best approach such situations involves utilizing problem-focused and emotion-focused coping.

Problem-Focused Coping

Problem-focused coping is ideal in circumstances when you can resolve stress through clear decision-making and direct action. These are situations best dealt with by gathering information, logically reviewing and analyzing the pros and cons, and then forming a plan—perhaps in the form of a to-do list.

Say you're choosing where to get your treatment. Problem-focused coping might involve looking into several different cancer centers, logically reviewing these options, and then analyzing the pros and cons of each. Ask yourself questions—"Which centers specialize in my type of cancer?" "Which are reasonably close to my home?"—and then make a plan of action to call the handful of best options on your list and schedule visits. To avoid feeling overwhelmed, try breaking down the project into smaller, workable steps. If you don't have the time or energy to drive to every center you're considering, you might arrange for informational Zoom calls with a couple of places or limit your choices to those centers within a certain number of miles.

The same approach can work in many other parts of treatment. Whether it's choosing which work or classes you may have to give up, setting boundaries with your family and friends around visits, or deciding when and how to ask for help, try to examine the situation carefully, ask yourself questions, listen to yourself, and focus on the plan.

In those cases where you don't have full control, problem-focused coping can still provide you with a sense of agency. Let's say you are experiencing nausea as a result of your treatment. Even if you can't totally eliminate the issue, you can take steps to address it. You can reach out to your doctor or nurse and say, "That regimen you gave me for post-chemo is not really treating my nausea as well as I'd like. Let's explore other options. Perhaps there is a different plan that might better control the nausea." Another regimen might work and it might not—but either way, you've taken some action to try to resolve or minimize the problem.

Emotion-Focused Coping

Emotion-focused coping is more useful when dealing with feelings of distress around painful, difficult situations or dilemmas that are *not* changeable. Since you can't problem-solve your way through them and change the situation, the healthiest approach is to find ways to acknowledge, accept, and manage your emotions.

This technique works in situations such as a cancer recurrence or the end of a relationship. Problems like these can't be stopped, but it may be conducive for you to process, channel, and express your emotions around them. That could involve talking with someone; finding ways to self-soothe, such as through meditation or spirituality; or getting your emotions out by journaling, drawing, or painting. Accepting does not mean you're *happy* with a situation or with how you are feeling, but talking about, examining, and processing your feelings can be beneficial—as difficult as this can be.

It is best to be flexible about whether to use problem-focused or emotion-focused coping, because most instances are not so clear-cut that only one technique applies. Having worked with cancer patients for more than thirty years, it is my experience that even when you feel like you're facing what seem like unchangeable circumstances, there are still some aspects of the situation—like with the chemo-related nausea—where problem-solving can be useful. Similarly, in instances when you are in full control, like choosing a cancer center, emotions can still play a role in your decision. Many people try to control situations, or even other people—but the reality is this: The only person you can actually work on directly is yourself. Learning how to self-manage, self-regulate, and self-soothe is vitally important for everyone.

Of course, this is easier said than done. Part of what can happen—and one of the reasons why emotion-focused coping is not always so easy—is that when you're faced with challenging and stressful situations, your emotions can feel overwhelming and terrifying. When you get extremely emotional, you can't think straight, especially in those instances where you feel threatened. This goes back to the fight-or-flight mode we discussed in Chapter 2. Remember, in terms of evolution, our bodies respond the same to a physical threat as to an emotional one. Split-second decisions need to be made. Rationally and calmly thinking through emotions is not an option in these moments, so we are left with these overwhelming, scary, and—yes, uncontrollable—emotions. Only later do we realize we may have behaved irrationally.

If these emotionally threatening instances involve other people, you may say or do things that you later regret. In other cases, you might just pull back and shut down. There is no easy answer, but self-soothing can help you to emotionally regulate in such situations. Learning these strategies actually often starts in childhood. A very simple example of self-soothing is when a baby is given a pacifier to pacify (or soothe) themselves. The hope is that as time goes on, the baby will find new soothing strategies when they feel upset, like grabbing a teddy bear, and will no longer need the pacifier.

This is a lifelong process. You will constantly be developing additional self-soothing strategies as you grow and have new experiences and interactions that you need to modulate. You may find that some of your old strategies, like that teddy bear, continue to work while others like the pacifier do not.

Start with the Basics

It is critical to include self-care as part of your daily life during and after your cancer treatment. But it may not be easy to figure out how. Since your daily life is likely already stressful enough, you may struggle trying to incorporate any of these ideas into it. On the other hand, perhaps because of all you've dealt with since your diagnosis, you might be more motivated to explore new activities and find new ways to manage your stress and emotions. Hopefully, that will be the case— you'll *want* to take better care of yourself. But just as with a New Year's resolution, it may be difficult to follow through on such actions during and beyond your treatment. If you find that to be the case, start with the basics and take small steps.

So, with this in mind, here is a closer look at the basics: eating healthy, staying hydrated, getting exercise, getting sleep, and trying to relax.

Eating Healthy

This seems like a no-brainer, but it's easy to get so busy that you don't really focus on healthy eating. Sometimes you may even notice a whole day has gone by, and you have not eaten at all! Or perhaps you ate some small, high-caloric, sugary treat that provided a quick burst of energy but then left you fatigued afterward. The key is learning not only how to eat healthy but how to make this your new lifestyle—not something short-term.

So what can you do? I often recommend to my patients that they go see one of our RDs (registered dietitians—see Chapter 4 for more on these professionals) trained to work with people in this exact situation.

An RD can help you devise a healthy eating plan that works for you—one that fits your schedule, is filled with foods you enjoy, and adheres to your cultural background and any allergies you may have. It's not an "all-or-none" approach. You can still occasionally enjoy chocolate or ice cream while eating healthy, because we know that denying ourselves things forever is not necessarily the way to go. It's really about *moderation*, and that's why I urge people to create a flexible approach and to make small gradual changes.

Staying Hydrated

Hydration is a major issue. If you are not drinking enough, you're going to feel fatigued and mentally foggy. It's no good to drink coffee all day instead of water either, because coffee just makes you urinate and become even *more* dehydrated. Whether you want to carry around a trendy bottle covered in stickers, flavor your water with fruit, or embrace a giant jug with timed goals printed on its side, find a way to drink enough water.

Getting Exercise

Everyone knows that exercise is good for your overall physical and mental health. It helps protect you against health problems; is a great means of combating anxiety, stress, and sadness; and is also good for your cognitive health.

The key, whether you're new to exercise, adjusting your level of activity during treatment, or resuming it after cancer treatment, is to start small. Find ways to incorporate more movement into your daily life. Park in the back of the parking lot so you have a longer walk to and from work. Go up and down extra flights of stairs in your home. Spend thirty seconds going "up-down-up-down" on a chair. Take a walk around the block, or even better, plan walks with friends so you have company and someone to hold you accountable.

Once you are feeling more energetic, consider taking up a new activity like yoga, pickleball, or swimming. If you're having trouble finding something, or feel intimidated, seek help from an organization used to working with people during and after cancer treatment. It makes no sense, nor is it helpful, to attend a yoga class geared to those who have *not* been through treatment. See if your cancer center has a physical therapist or exercise physiologist who will meet with you for an evaluation. Once they see your capabilities, they can devise programs for you to do on your own as well as connect you with classes designed specifically for people at different stages of their cancer trajectory. Be sure to ask for both.

Patient Voices

"Navigating a cancer diagnosis and years of treatment can be incredibly stressful and draining, until you realize that you have the power to control your reactions. The most important thing is to find joy in every new day (for me, it's either through dance, yoga, or cooking a nice meal). Taking care of my mind through daily meditations and taking care of my body through daily exercise have been crucial for my healing process, and has also helped boost the effectiveness of treatments." —Orsolya K.

Getting Sleep

Try to get seven to eight hours of sleep a night. Again, this is easy to suggest but can be difficult to implement. During treatment, you may lose your regular sleep schedule. Side effects can interfere with your sleep. Worrying may not allow you to fall or stay asleep. Some suggestions you could try include:

- Developing a bedtime routine, including a specific time to go to sleep and wake up
- Using your bed only for sleep (and sex)
- Keeping your bedroom cool
- Minimizing daytime sleeping
- Avoiding use of your phone or laptop in bed
- Trying to fall asleep before midnight
- Avoiding caffeine and exercise close to bedtime

- Using relaxation techniques before bedtime (see next section)
- Writing out your next day's to-do list before bed
- Setting aside thirty minutes daily to focus on your worrying thoughts, so you don't take them to bed
- Getting out of bed after thirty minutes if you're not asleep and only going back when sleepy

I also often ask patients to keep a sleep diary for five days, noting the time they go to bed, the time they fall asleep, and the time they wake up. The Resources section lists some options to help with insomnia.

Relaxation Techniques

A great way of reducing stress is finding ways to bring about your body's relaxation response, which is characterized by slower breathing, lower blood pressure, and a reduced heart rate. One method that works well for a lot of people is diaphragmatic breathing (or belly breathing). If you want to give this a try, set aside a few minutes at the same time each day to practice—so that it becomes a regular part of your routine.

Here's what belly breathing entails:

1. Find a quiet place so as to minimize external distractions.
2. Lie down on a recliner or couch, or on the floor with your back propped up by pillows.
3. Place one hand on your chest and one hand on your belly.
4. Put on a soothing and relaxing song (most songs last for about two to three and half minutes).
5. Breathe normally, in and out through your nose, for the length of the song. Focus on bringing each breath all the way down through your diaphragm to your belly, noticing that when you breathe in, it is your belly getting distended—not your chest. Only the hand on your belly should move.
6. Repeat daily, ideally as part of your bedtime routine.

While this sounds easy, it can actually be quite challenging. Your mind will wander, and you'll notice that you are breathing shallowly and only your chest is moving. That's okay; just try and refocus on your belly.

Another great relaxation technique is thirty-second mindfulness, which I will explain shortly when we talk about mindfulness.

Adding to the Basics

Self-care is more than taking time now and then for a manicure, pedicure, or massage. Sure, pampering can help, but you need to incorporate self-care as *part of your daily life*, because, as we've talked about, stress can be part of your life with cancer from the moment you wake up.

The following lists offer a variety of possible methods you can use to regulate and manage your emotions and stress level on a daily basis during and after cancer treatment. Everyone is different, so it's important you find what works for you. Keep in mind that this list is not exhaustive—it's just some ideas to get you started.

Remember, if you're not doing well physically, that will have an impact on all aspects of your life. It's the same if you're not at your best *mentally*—that can then affect the physical and social aspects of your life. It's all interconnected, and everything impacts everything else. When you engage in an activity that helps your physical well-being, such as taking a yoga class, it can also brighten your mood. If you meet other people while there, that adds a social component, and you may even find that the relaxation exercise at the end of the yoga class provides a spiritual component. Ideally, you will be able to utilize some or several of these approaches to impact and create a ripple effect across the different facets of your mental health. This list opens with the basics as a gentle reminder, then gives you dozens of ideas to try.

The Basics
- Healthy eating and regularly hydrating
- Physical activity and exercise
- Sleep (seven to eight hours nightly)

Additional Ideas—Add to the Basics

- Time with pets (consider adopting your own)
- Connecting with nature (through walks, visiting parks, or sitting outside)
- Meditation and mindfulness (start with belly breathing)
- Warm baths or showers
- Daily gratitude practice

Art/Education

- Doodling, drawing, and/or painting
- Collaging (using old magazines and newspapers)
- Scrapbooking
- Ceramics and jewelry making
- Taking photos and/or videos around your community
- Museum visits to appreciate art, history, science, etc.
- Learning a new language (at home or in a class)
- Taking classes (virtually or in person)

Writing/Reading

- Keeping a gratitude journal
- Expressing feelings in a diary (to share or keep to yourself)
- Writing poetry
- Creative writing
- Therapeutic journaling (consider trying the Pennebaker Writing Protocol to process your emotions)
- Joining a book club
- Reading or listening to audiobooks

Music/Dance/Theater

- Listening to music and creating playlists
- Writing your own music
- Playing instruments (or learning a new one)
- Singing (by yourself or in a choir)
- Learning to dance (or taking a new dance class)

- Dancing for fun at home
- Attending theater, opera, or improv shows
- Joining a theater or improv group (or creating your own)
- Seeking out a professional expressive arts therapist to guide you through different forms of art as a way of expressing and processing your emotions (your oncology team can help you find one)

Games/Humor
- Video gaming (alone or in online groups)
- Board games with friends
- Puzzles
- Funny movies or YouTube and TikTok videos
- Joke and humor books
- Dark humor (for helping to cope with cancer)
- Anything silly or fun (and safe) that gives you pleasure

Hobbies
- Cooking
- Gardening
- Bird-watching
- Thrifting
- Knitting or crocheting or embroidery
- Watching or going to movies
- Traveling (within the limits of your treatment)
- Shopping or window shopping on the Internet

Spirituality and Faith
- Attending religious services or gatherings
- Praying anywhere (to help soothe or calm yourself)
- Joining a faith-based group or retreat
- Volunteering with organizations aligned with your values, such as houses of worship, shelters, hospitals, or museums (before volunteering with others undergoing cancer treatment, wait until a year after finishing your own treatment)

- Advocating locally or nationally for a worthy cause (perhaps cancer funding)
- Delivering meals to people who are sick or in mourning, as part of a "meal train"

Most of the ideas listed are fairly self-explanatory. Here's some additional information and tips to help you dive into some of them:

- **Expressive writing:** In terms of expressing and connecting with your emotions, as well as processing them, expressive writing (therapeutic journaling) can be very helpful. Research has shown it can lead to reductions in stress and anxiety. Just write out your feelings, without editing or judging your thoughts, when you're feeling emotionally overwhelmed. You can keep the finished product or throw it out; the value is in doing it.
- **Art and music:** Like writing, art and music are ways to get feelings out. I often encourage patients to do things like "draw out your anger" or "paint your sadness." Music can also aid you in connecting with your feelings and even in changing your mood. Songs you listen to (or play yourself) can bring back vivid memories and feelings of particular moments or times, and/or soothe or energize you. Other forms of art, including dancing and theater, can also help you to express—and explore—your feelings. Keep in mind that you don't have to be artistic to explore any of this. It is not about the product you produce, but about the process you are engaging in.

Managing Change and Equilibrium

There are other things besides daily stressors and trying to do too much too soon that can interfere with your continuing to engage in the stress-management and self-soothing tactics we've discussed thus far. Initially, you may be so happy and relieved after completing active treatment that you're excited simply to enjoy simple pleasures that you've missed, such as eating well or going on walks. You want stability. People who have reached this point will often say to me, "I don't want anything eventful. I just want things to go easily and smoothly." They are *thrilled* with stability.

What you may find as time goes on, however, is that you start to notice that you are no longer feeling as good with that stability. You start to become dissatisfied and bothered by little things. As human beings, we always go back to a place of equilibrium, whether physiologically or emotionally. So while initially something might make you really happy, you adjust to that happiness over time and gradually creep back into equilibrium. The same happens for sad events. You may feel a great deal of anguish after a loss, but over time—while you will still likely feel sadness—you go back to a state of equilibrium where the grief is not as intense.

This also helps to explain the social media technique by which a "dopamine rush" (e.g., a new item or exciting experience) provides temporary happiness. Psychologists have come up with the term "hedonic treadmill" to describe how we are constantly looking for that next thrill we want to feel.

This phenomenon is why, if you work out with a personal trainer, they will frequently advise you to "change things up." Do yoga one day, weight training another day, and maybe basketball or running the day after that. By keeping things interesting, and different, the trainer hopes to keep you better engaged. When you try new activities, particularly with other people, it seems to have a lasting effect. The more memorable the experiences, the more likely you are to revisit them and feel that happiness again.

That's why our list of possible self-care activities is so long—because hopefully you will try one thing, and then another, and then something else. Whether you learn a new language or a new instrument, you'll find ways to keep yourself engaged. Whatever you try, make an effort to really *enjoy* it and see what it's all about. You don't have to be good at it; this is not about achievement but about jumping in and focusing on experiencing something new.

Incorporating Mindfulness

I routinely have patients come back to me for tune-ups after completing their initial therapy. When I ask them why, they tell me, "You know, for the first few months after I finished treatment, I was constantly excited about learning new things. I kept up with your suggestions and was taking all the steps that I thought were important for my general health and well-being. But as time goes by, I'm starting to get upset by trivial everyday occurrences. I know this doesn't make sense, but I'm getting just as bothered by things as I did before the cancer."

Why is this happening to them? I think that initially—and understandably—people are thrilled to be done with cancer treatment and feel more in control of their lives again. But then, as that equilibrium sets in and things return to more of a balanced, normal state, they find themselves looking to get that feeling of constant happiness back. We know that it is impossible to feel happy all the time, but we also know that if you're *looking* for happiness all the time, you're missing the day-to-day experiences that might bring you unexpected joy. That saying, "Stop and smell the roses" may be a platitude, but it really is true.

This is where mindfulness comes in. Engaging in mindfulness is one very important way to keep a daily focus on what is happening in your life and how you are experiencing it. Mindfulness is the practice of noticing your thoughts, emotions, and experiences in the present moment, without judgment. That's a simple definition, but it's quite hard to accomplish. It does not mean just to *clear* your mind; that's a misconception. What it's really about is *being aware*.

Thirty-Second Mindfulness Exercise

Here's an easy way to gradually start bringing mindfulness into your life:

1. Pick an activity that offers the opportunity to use an abundance of your senses—smell, touch/feel, temperature, sight, taste, hearing. For example, sitting outside in a garden is ideal for this exercise.

2. Set a timer for thirty seconds.
3. Start the timer and try to focus on all your senses.
   - What do you *smell*? The flowers? The air?
   - Take a moment to touch and notice how things *feel*. Feel the leaves, or the ground, or the temperature. Feel the sun or breeze on your face.
   - Now focus on your *sight*. Are there flowers blooming or leaves of all different, vibrant colors, or is there snow on the ground? Look up. Are there clouds in the sky? Is it blue? Is it overcast?
   - Then take in the *sounds*. What do you hear? The birds chirping? The leaves rustling? The wind blowing? Children laughing down the street?
4. Set aside thirty seconds every day to seek out your senses.
   - Consider changing location and/or activity.

It's all about being mindful for those thirty seconds. You can apply it to anything, as long as you keep it novel and new. Perhaps you're eating a special meal you took time to prepare and are excited to eat. How does it smell? How does it look? Put it in your mouth and feel its warmth. How does it taste?

Or maybe you're reading a book with your child or sitting next to your partner. Whatever the activity, try and take it in with all your senses. What does your child or partner smell like? Put your arm around them. What do they feel like? What do they look like? What are you hearing as you read to them or sit beside them? The activity itself might last five, ten, or twenty minutes, but thirty seconds is all you need to really *experience* the moment through mindfulness. In the future, you might gradually increase the time you spend on this exercise and try sixty seconds and then maybe ninety seconds.

Patient Voices

"The cancer diagnosis shocked me to face the deeply uncomfortable yet universal truth that life is finite. During

treatment, I found myself with ample time to be still and think. I tried mindfulness for a few minutes a day and discovered that being present offered a refreshing reprieve from the constant cycle of dwelling on the past or being concerned with the future. Physically, it helped me be more attuned with my body, and mentally, it brought my attention to the positive things around me." —Darren C.

Practice Mindfulness with Gratitude Journaling

Gratitude is an emotion that involves feeling thankful for the good things in your life. It can come from a general sense of appreciation for what is meaningful and/or from the direct act of giving and receiving. In terms of overall well-being, gratitude is associated with better mental health, improved self-esteem, less stress, better sleep, improved relationships, and a greater ability to cope with adversity. People who practice a life focused on gratitude also tend to be more altruistic.

Gratitude journaling involves mindfully writing each day about one (or three) thing(s) for which you are truly grateful. It can't be something general, like, "I'm thankful for my health." It has to be specific: "Today I'm thankful that my energy was better, and I was able to climb an extra flight of stairs." Try doing it every day for a year, and then review it (it's okay if you miss some days). You will be surprised how your year will no longer feel like a blur when you can look to your journal and remember specific days—and the joys you experienced on them.

It's not always easy to be grateful. This is especially true when facing challenges or trying to achieve unrealistic expectations you may have set for yourself. Due to other interfering emotions, such as envy and cynicism, gratitude comes easier for some than others. I have always thought that those who struggle with gratitude, and look at situations (or people) in black-and-white terms—all good versus all bad— will have a more difficult time in life. With practice, though, I believe we can *all* feel more gratitude and be mindful about what's going well in our lives.

It's Okay to Be Distracted

Sometimes a patient will say to me, "Ugh, I just spent a whole day mindlessly doing things like binging a show and distracting myself." Well, that serves a function too. Sometimes you simply don't have the energy to be engrossed in or fully mindful of anything substantive. So you "mindlessly" get engaged in something like doodling. That's okay. If, in the end, you enjoyed yourself, the time was valuable. You can watch a sitcom and look at it as either distraction or humor—and you're engaged in it by laughing. So it's really not so much about the activities you do but rather *how you approach them* and what function they serve for you at a given moment.

Mindfulness Meditation

Research suggests that meditation is very beneficial for your overall well-being, including helping with stress reduction, emotional regulation, pain management, and (in conjunction with other approaches) anxiety and depression. There are different types of meditation practices. Mindfulness meditation is a type of practice in which you focus on your breath and your body to cultivate a state of being mindful. There is no *right* type of meditation; whatever works for you is the correct choice. When choosing a practice, however, it is helpful to either use an app or work with someone who can guide you through the process. There are plenty of great mindfulness apps out there to explore, and many cancer centers and other facilities offer meditation classes led by experts in the field.

Pets As Stress Reducers

I am a huge proponent of pets and the meaningful role that they can provide in your life—including during cancer treatment. There is a great deal of research showing that touching and stroking a pet can lower your stress levels and help reduce anxiety and sadness. A pet can also provide wonderful companionship to help you cope during trying times, and get you outside for regular exercise and the chance to form social connections. Taking your dog for a walk not only keeps you moving, but if you head to a dog park—or even just stroll around your neighborhood—there is a good chance you'll meet people with whom you already have something important in common.

The benefits are there even if the pet is not yours. Dog therapy programs in hospitals help patients feel less anxious and stressed. The staff usually enjoys interacting with the dogs, so they give them a real boost as well. Throughout the years, I've suggested my young adult patients consider getting a pet. I also practice what I preach. Zoe, my miniature dachshund, is my constant companion. She is with me—usually on my lap—when I'm at work or meeting with patients virtually.

In addition to extolling the benefits of lap animals, I also suggest patients consider horse-assisted therapy—which can be very helpful in teaching emotional regulation (or the ability to manage your emotions). Because horses respond to our emotions and heart rates, you need to communicate calmly with them—especially when riding. If you are stressed out, or your heart rate increases, or your mood changes, a horse will feel it and give you pretty immediate feedback, usually by picking up its pace and not being as responsive to your commands. That reaction can help you learn to regulate your emotions, whether on a horse or (hopefully) in navigating the ups and downs of your cancer trajectory.

Key Points

- Your mental health is as important as your physical health. Self-care activities can help you properly maintain your mental health during and after treatment.
- Stress and difficult emotions are a normal part of the cancer trajectory. Learning to manage stress and identify and process emotions will help you to better cope with each new stage and challenge.

- For both your mental and physical health, be sure to eat well, get enough sleep, exercise (start small!), and stay hydrated.
- There are endless ways to practice self-care during your treatment. From time in nature to creative writing to pet therapy, try some options that excite you, and change them up from time to time.
- Mindfulness—or focusing on the present moment without judgment—is a valuable way to reduce stress, relax, and recognize and appreciate what's around you.

CHAPTER 7
Psychotherapy As Part of Treatment

Cindy was diagnosed with breast cancer just after turning thirty, but in some ways she felt like she had been waiting years for the news.

Her maternal grandmother had died of ovarian cancer when Cindy was little, her maternal aunt had died in her mid-forties from breast cancer, and her mom was a breast cancer survivor. Cindy figured it was only a matter of time until her family's genetic history caught up to her.

Reconnecting with a psychologist she had seen to help manage her anxiety during college, Cindy learned how to help herself emotionally regulate as she faced this new challenge. She engaged in mindful meditation twice daily and, after years of sporadic exercise, finally began a consistent, disciplined workout program. Her therapist emphasized how strong social support is a key to good mental health—especially during trying times—so Cindy also made a conscious effort to go out more with friends.

Once she completed chemotherapy, surgery, and radiation, Cindy expected she would start feeling better. Instead, she found herself ruminating, worrying, and sweating so badly that it took her hours each night to fall asleep. This, naturally, led to extreme fatigue.

"I began losing my concentration at work, something that had never happened before," says Cindy. "When I looked in the mirror, I didn't even feel like I was looking at myself because of all the physical changes. It was like I was still in treatment."

Cindy shared some of her frustration with her nurse practitioner and was referred to me for treatment. During our first meeting, we discussed how even though she had finished chemotherapy, she was still on "active" treatment to try to prevent breast cancer from recurring. This treatment had caused her to be in premature menopause, with some of the related side effects, including treatment-related fatigue, cognitive issues, weight gain, and night sweats as well as sleep and emotional changes.

Because Cindy was to continue this regimen for at least five years to help prevent her breast cancer from returning, we discussed different coping strategies as well as possible referrals to other providers, such as integrative medicine and psychiatry professionals, to help her manage the side effects. Some antidepressants, I explained to her, have been shown to help with hot flashes, sleep issues, and other premature menopause symptoms, while acupuncture and exercise could also aid in sleep issues, hot flashes, and joint pain associated with her treatment.

"Therapy helped me develop ways to respond to people who expected me to feel and function like I did before cancer, such as explaining to them that my current medication, while an oral treatment, is powerful just like my chemo was," says Cindy. "I also gained a new understanding of how my family history related to my current situation. Even though I had long known my chances for getting cancer were higher, I had never really worked through how this knowledge might have affected me growing up."

The Importance of Professional Support

While some of you are aware of or have experienced the benefits of seeing a mental health professional (MHP), others may never have considered it. The thought of sitting with an MHP can be frightening. You may wonder, "How could they help me anyway? I still have cancer. Why would I want to talk with a stranger about my most intimate thoughts and feelings?" The misrepresentations we see in the media of MHPs being "crazy" themselves don't help, either.

In reality, most MHPs specializing in oncology are fairly typical human beings who have chosen to train and work in a field where they can try and help those with cancer to better deal with and navigate this extremely challenging time. MHPs in psychosocial oncology focus on providing psycho-education, support, validation of your feelings and experiences, and specific strategies to cope with cancer and cancer treatment, as well as connect you with local and national resources. At times, simply being able to talk through your feelings with an MHP gives you clarity and perspective. You can share your emotions and thoughts without being judged—and without having to worry about upsetting them. This makes psychotherapy pretty unique, because the focus is on *you* and not the other person.

As a clinical psychologist, I tend to feel that *everyone* can benefit from psychotherapy. I will often suggest to patients who express hesitancy to give it a try and meet with me one time before refusing outright. I do understand that for some of you, due to your upbringing and/or culture, speaking to your clergy (or a specific support person) may feel more "right"—which I totally support. I often see young adults who also regularly meet with their clergy, or even continue seeing a prior therapist who does *not* specialize in psychosocial oncology. I hope this chapter illustrates the specific ways that MHPs in psychosocial oncology can be of assistance throughout and beyond your cancer course.

Situations to Be Aware Of

While everyone experiences a spectrum of feelings during their cancer trajectories, sometimes the symptoms can become more severe and interfere with your ability to function. Following is a list of specific times when referral to a mental health professional is especially important. **If you know or believe any of these circumstances apply to you, please seek a referral from your clinical team to a mental health professional:**

- Risk of harm to yourself or others
- Depression and/or anxiety interfering with functioning

- History of major mental illness and/or substance use
- Family history of major mental illness and/or substance use
- Indecision about treatment and/or treatment options
- History of panic attacks and/or phobias (e.g., needle phobia, claustrophobia, generalized anxiety)
- Sexual difficulties or sexual changes resulting from cancer treatment
- Other stressors concurrent with your cancer (e.g., death of a parent, spouse, or child; divorce/breakup; job loss)
- Being pregnant when diagnosed and/or during treatment
- Perceived lack of social support
- Family, marital, or relationship problems interfering with treatment
- Conflict between you, your family, and the medical staff

Major Depression

Some of the situations listed here are self-explanatory, while others are harder to decipher. If you have previously been diagnosed with depression, your cancer diagnosis and treatment may cause a relapse or exacerbate existing symptoms. For this reason, it is essential that your cancer treatment team know about your depression *from the start*, so that they can connect you with the right resources to minimize the likelihood of a relapse, as well as treat any existing symptoms.

In addition, cancer patients face the possibility of major depression if they have a history of depression. "Depression" is a broad term that encompasses various degrees of low moods, while major depression (also known as major depressive disorder or clinical depression) is a specific form. Diagnosing major depression during or after cancer treatment is tricky because so many of the symptoms associated with major depression and cancer treatments are the same—including problems with sleeping and concentrating and drops in appetite and energy. Often mental health professionals working in oncology will also consider other symptoms that are not easily influenced by cancer treatment to help make the diagnosis of major depression; these may include excessive, uncontrollable crying; increased irritability; extreme ruminating on negative thoughts; feelings of worthlessness; and indecision.

Meeting with a mental health professional can also really help tease out what's going on. In my experience, young adults with cancer who don't meet the full criteria for major depression might still benefit from therapy. Such a step can help you develop the tools needed to cope with cancer, especially with so much else going on in your life.

Rates of major depression are higher in young adults with cancer than in their older counterparts. Some common variables associated with the increased risk include a history (personal or family) of depression, a history (personal or family) of alcohol and/or substance use, a recurrent/advanced cancer with higher symptom burden, decreased physical abilities, poorly managed pain, and a higher risk for suicide (seventeen- to thirty-nine-year-olds with cancer are at increased risk compared to same-age peers without a cancer diagnosis).

Increased Anxiety

Most young adults will experience some anxiety and worry throughout their treatment courses. But some situations—such as a personal or family history of anxiety disorder, the presence of certain brain or gland tumors, poorly managed pain, steroid medications, and a cancer recurrence—can raise the chance for heightened anxiety that interferes with functioning. If you have any of those risk factors, consider requesting additional resources and assistance with anxiety.

Cancer Treatments Can Affect Your Mood

Your oncologist is focused on treating your cancer and may not necessarily concentrate on the psychiatric side effects of certain cancer treatments. If you notice major emotional changes while undergoing treatment, consider referring to the following list of medications to see if any you are on may be affecting your mood:

- Keppra (levetiracetam)—associated with irritability, anxiety, aggression, and depression
- Some chemotherapy and immunotherapy can be associated with anxiety, depression, sleep changes, fatigue, appetite changes, and/or concentration difficulties:
  - Ifosfamide
  - Interferon-alpha—associated with anxiety
  - Interleukin-2
  - Ipilimumab
  - L-asparaginase
  - Nivolumab
  - Pembrolizumab
  - Procarbazine
  - Steroids (decadron and prednisone)—associated with anxiety, sleep disturbance, depression, irritability, and aggression
  - Tamoxifen and aromatase inhibitors
  - Temozolomide—associated with depression and anxiety
  - Vinblastine
  - Vincristine

If you notice these symptoms while on any of these medicines, advocate for yourself and ask to see a psychiatrist trained in psycho-social oncology. They can help you manage any mood changes you experience, since you may not be able to—or want to—stop the cancer medication causing them.

Finding the Right Therapist for You

Just as when you looked for an oncologist, it is important to try to find a therapist who's a good fit for you and your situation. You need to feel comfortable with the person. Given that this individual will be with you through such a trying time, you want to feel they are empathic and understanding. I also strongly recommend you give preference to therapists who possess the specialized training needed to work with cancer patients and families—or, if not trained in cancer specifically, are at least well versed in medical or health conditions in general. As you'll see in this section, there are many reasons for making this a point of consideration.

Different Types of Therapists

Mental health professionals have varied levels of training. These are the three primary types of therapists you will likely encounter in your treatment—and who you may want to seek out on your own:

- A **social worker** typically has a four-year undergraduate degree and a master's in social work (MSW) degree requiring two additional years of advanced training. Both licensed clinical social workers (LCSWs) and licensed independent social workers (LISWs) must pass a national exam, complete a period of supervised experience, and possess an MSW degree.
- A **clinical psychologist** must have a doctor of philosophy (PhD) or doctor of psychology (PsyD) degree, each of which requires at least six years of training beyond a standard four-year undergraduate degree. Only practitioners with a doctorate can call themselves "psychologists"—and they always must be licensed by the state they practice in.
- A **psychiatrist** needs to have a doctor of medicine (MD) or doctor of osteopathic medicine (DO) degree. Both require at least seven years of education and training beyond an undergraduate degree. Psychiatrists may, after their residency, decide to complete a fellowship specializing in working with medically ill patients—including those with cancer. Of the therapists listed here, only a psychiatrist can prescribe medicine. Psychiatrists have specialized training in psychopharmacology: a distinct understanding of how medications move through the body and interact with different drugs, and the impact that each person's specific genetic makeup can play in their response to medication.

All of these professionals may also choose to seek a fellowship in psychosocial oncology, which requires one or two years of additional training. A psychosocial oncology fellowship is a huge commitment in time and energy and not something every mental health professional will undertake, but there is clearly a need for more therapists with cancer-specific knowledge and training. There are continuing education programs such as the one offered at Dana-Farber—in conjunction with Harvard Medical School—for those therapists who are seeing cancer patients and families in their practice but are unable to commit to formal, comprehensive fellowship training. "Therapist" is a very general term and can refer to any of the previously listed MHPs as well as to other people who may not be licensed and trained to work as an MHP. When seeking mental health support, proceed cautiously and inquire about training and state licensure.

Patient Voices

"I've learned that it's okay to 'date' a few therapists before finding the right one. I was in therapy during treatment but remember still feeling alone. You don't have to feel bad for ghosting a therapist who isn't the right fit—it took me three tries to find mine. Therapy gave me tools, like breathing exercises to ease weekly panic attacks. More than that, it helped me feel safe in my own skin again and embrace the new version of myself with compassion." —Aaidaliz P.

The Benefits of a Cancer-Trained Therapist

I suggest that any mental health professional you see be trained in psychosocial oncology, either through a fellowship (ideally) or by training at a cancer center. Therapists without such training often lack a complete understanding of the cancer journey and won't be able to give you specific insight or treatment that's tailored to your situation. While they may *mean* well, their advice could be confusing or potentially even incorrect.

Here are several key reasons that a mental health provider trained in cancer treatment is especially valuable.

They Understand Cancer Treatment Medications

Your mental health provider should be familiar with the many different cancer medications you are taking or might be prescribed, as well as knowledgeable in how these drugs may impact you physically and psychologically.

One situation in which this misdiagnosis can happen is when dealing with steroids. Steroids are prescribed for a wide variety of reasons during cancer treatment, and high doses of steroids commonly interfere with sleep as well as cause irritability, anger, anxiety, and agitation in cancer patients. Having a therapist who knows to look for such responses can be critical in your mental health treatment.

For instance, I once was referred to a patient whose wife assured me was typically quite mild mannered and easygoing but had recently begun angrily yelling and throwing things (even furniture!) at home. I suspected that high doses of steroids might be the reason, especially when the patient described to me how he struggled to sit still, was irritable, and couldn't manage his emotions. The patient's oncology team confirmed that he had indeed been on very high doses of steroids for a prolonged period, and that these were likely contributing to his difficulties. A therapist not trained in cancer medications might have just assumed the patient's strong emotional changes were the result of being too stressed or marital communication problems. My cancer knowledge was very helpful in making this assessment, and in working with the patient and their family to develop coping strategies.

They Can Address Concerns of Addiction

Most cancer patients do not become addicts from taking prescribed pain medication for their cancer-related pain. Yet, many patients are very *concerned* about becoming addicted, even if they have never had this problem in the past. A psychosocial oncology professional can help alleviate such concerns by working with the oncology team to educate these patients that the medications in question are prescribed appropriately to treat their pain.

Similarly, when there are legitimate fears of addiction due to a patient's past substance use, an experienced mental health professional will know how to closely partner with the patient's oncology team—and involve pain management and palliative care teams as needed—to make sure the individual's pain is managed and alleviated while concerns related to their prior substance use are also addressed.

They Use a Family-Centered Approach

While mental health treatment is typically individualized and patient-centered therapy, when it involves cancer patients—particularly young adults—an individual's family will often need to be involved and educated about what's going on. A family-centered approach is frequently necessary, as illustrated in the steroid rage situation described earlier. In such instances, the patient's spouse, partner, or primary caregiver needs to be educated as to why the patient is so angry or behaving irrationally.

They Recognize and Respect Bodily Changes

Therapists lacking oncology experience may also not be accustomed to some of the bodily changes that cancer patients go through. It is not unusual, for instance, for someone to say to me, "I've had breast reconstruction and I'm not so happy with how it looks." By virtue of my background I have books I can share and discuss filled with photos of different breast reconstructions, so they can compare their appearance with others.

Cancer treatment can impact your body in numerous ways beyond surgery, of course. When it comes to two of the most unpredictable and embarrassing—throwing up and passing gas—mental health professionals with a background treating cancer patients are understanding and are accustomed to such situations. They will likely know to have a trash bucket and nearby bathroom ready and a water bottle ready to offer. Even if you can't help but feel uncomfortable during such moments, it's great to have a therapist who reacts to them with a caring hand rather than awkwardness.

Similarly, a therapist familiar with the challenges of cancer treatment will recognize you are not always going to feel well from one day to the next. They will know there are times you might need help standing up or sitting down at therapy. And while many mental health professionals will charge you in full for a missed session if you're too sick to come—and not let you cancel less than twenty-four hours beforehand—a cancer-conscious therapist is apt to cut you some slack and let you reschedule free of charge. Considering all the costs that can come your way during your cancer trajectory, this kind of empathy is great to have. They can accommodate a shorter session when necessary if you are too fatigued. If you are hospitalized, they can see you as an inpatient because they usually have hospital privileges and they understand the importance of continuity of care across care settings.

How Psychological Treatment for Cancer Patients Usually Works

The model for psychological treatment for cancer patients focuses on the here and now, and brings in past experiences only when they impact and relate to what's going on during an individual's cancer treatment. Your initial meeting with a psychosocial oncology therapist will typically be very thorough: You will be asked how you are feeling presently, how you are dealing with your cancer, as well as about any past trauma, prior experiences with psychotherapy, and medications you may have taken for mental health concerns. In future sessions, however, your therapist will likely refer back to this information only if they deem it helpful to your current situation. The primary focus of your work together is helping you best deal with your cancer diagnosis and treatment.

I usually subscribe to this model, in that I do not typically discuss a patient's childhood or adolescence with them after their initial intake session unless I believe it is directly impacting and interfering with the patient's ability to access cancer treatment and/or function in a healthy way during it. When such a scenario *is* the case, and a patient's formative experiences might provide insight into their current state of mind—or behavior—it can be very useful to reexamine the past to help work through the present. Here's an example:

I was referred to a cancer patient who was forty-five, doing well, and happy with her job and family. During our intake session, she brought up that she had been sexually assaulted while in college. She told me she had worked through the ordeal with a trauma specialist but wanted to let me know just so that I was aware of it. As time went on, and we continued meeting, she went through her chemotherapy and surgery, did very well, and was scheduled to start radiation therapy.

Then something unexpected happened. As she lay alone on the radiation table for the first time and waited for the procedure to start, she suddenly felt very cold. During the radiation process, several minutes in which she had to remain completely still, she had a sensation of being restrained and out of control. As a sexual assault survivor, she was brought back to that trauma through this new experience—so in that case, the patient's past was very relevant to what was going on in her current treatment, and had to be dealt with as part of our therapy. Other examples of how the past may be relevant to the present include patients with a family history of cancer, a genetic predisposition to cancer, and other medical or genetic predispositions.

The story also illustrates another aspect of psychotherapy during and after cancer treatment: It is a crisis intervention model. In more typical outpatient psychotherapy, there may be more focus on reviewing a patient's childhood, while psychosocial oncology therapy tends to center on the cancer experience and how it impacts your life *now*—and in the future. The acknowledgment is that a crisis can occur at any point during a person's cancer trajectory, from diagnosis to treatment to post-treatment. In fact, it is often a series of crises, interspersed with intervals of relief and stability.

An effective cancer psychotherapist should be able to help you:

- **Clarify misconceptions and misinformation** about diagnosis, prognosis, and treatment (including medications), in consultation with your oncology team.

- **Reduce anxiety and distress** related to your diagnosis, treatment, and side effects, along with concurrent changes in your relationships, work life, and social life.
- **Decrease your feelings of isolation** through psycho-education and referral to group therapy and support groups.
- **Develop new coping strategies**, as well as utilize those that have worked for you in the past, to deal with your cancer experience and its ramifications.
- **Provide an overview at the end of the initial session** (and periodically going forward) of how they can help with specific recommendations, frequency of visits, referrals, and your agreement with the treatment suggestions.
- **Address and explore existential questions**, such as: "What is life all about?"; "What is the meaning of life in general, and for me?"; and "How do I want to live my life?"

We'll take a deeper dive into some of these topics next.

Group Therapy Options

Social isolation is a real challenge for early onset cancer patients. Young adult support and psycho-educational groups are a valuable way to address that concern. Such groups are important for social connection and give you a chance to talk with other young adults with cancer—who you may *not* encounter at other points of your treatment.

What Happens in Group Meetings

Seeing and conversing with your oncology peers can provide a strong sense of validation around what you're feeling, and while the thought of joining an in-person or virtual group can initially be somewhat intimidating, remember that you can always take it slow. You don't even necessarily need to participate in the discussion right away. Maybe start out by just listening, and then, as you feel more comfortable, consider joining in.

A critically important aspect of these group is the presence of a facilitator who is a credentialed mental health provider. Trained therapists are skilled at moderating sessions, keeping discussions on track, and making sure that everybody who wants to share has a chance to do so.

To help increase participation and allow people to get to know each other better, a facilitator might break up a large group into two or three smaller ones—which can be done virtually using "breakout rooms"—for more intimate discussions. At the end of my online groups, I like to leave the virtual chat open and let people stay on later and talk. My hope is that this simulates what used to happen when groups met in person, and participants would chat as they headed out at the end of sessions.

Different Types of Groups to Consider

There are many types of groups to seek out, depending on what you believe will work best for you. If you're not sure, ask your mental health provider or oncology team for their thoughts, or try different groups to find the best fit. And if your cancer center doesn't offer the type of group you're looking for, see if they can refer you—or reach out to one of the organizations listed in the Resources section.

One recent development that has dramatically increased the number of available options is the growth of virtual groups, which have now become the norm. You no longer need to worry about traveling to a session if you're fatigued or live far away; even those groups that still meet in person often have a hybrid option so that people can participate virtually.

Here are some of the different groups to consider, both for you and those in your life:

- Young adults newly diagnosed with cancer
- Young adults in active treatment
- Young adults in post-treatment
- Young adults with a site-specific cancer (e.g., young adults with breast cancer)
- Partners of young adults with cancer
- Parents of young adults with cancer

In addition to the theme or composition of the group, there are other options to consider, such as:

- **Time-limited versus ongoing groups:** A time-limited group lasts for a set number of sessions (often six to eight) and is structured so that there is a specific topic discussed each time. You may see a large percentage of the same people from session to session, as folks commit to attending a certain number. If you want less structure, however, other groups are ongoing, meeting weekly or monthly, with different people coming in and out all the time.
- **Structured skills versus support groups:** Structured skills groups tend to be organized, focusing on specific topics as a way of providing education along with support. Some examples include a journaling group, a group to learn stress management skills, a music therapy group, or an art therapy group. Support groups, in contrast, are less structured and don't have specific goals for each session. The objective is simply to meet participants where they are at, helping them with whatever concerns or issues they care to share.

Clearly, there are myriad types of group therapy to consider. You can review the options with your mental health provider and decide which one might be right for you.

Specific Therapeutic Approaches

Effective psychotherapy can help you both use those coping strategies that have worked for you in the past as well as develop new strategies to deal with your cancer and its ramifications. What follows are a few examples of specific therapeutic approaches.

Cognitive Behavioral Therapy

There is a great deal of research support for the effectiveness of cognitive behavioral therapy (CBT) to help with anxiety, depression, and other mental health conditions, and CBT is routinely used in psychosocial oncology care. It is a structured, symptom-focused, and collaborative approach. You and the therapist work closely together, and you have homework exercises between sessions.

The goal with CBT is to learn coping techniques that you can then use on your own. For example, the therapist will work with you to recognize your thoughts and cognitions and how they impact your feelings and behaviors. By identifying unhelpful thought patterns and learning how to modify them when necessary, you can start to regulate your feelings and emotions. A CBT therapist can also help you develop new problem-solving techniques, like setting aside worry time, behavioral activation, and diaphragmatic breathing. When it comes to phobias, anxiety, and/or panic attacks, CBT approaches including visualization techniques, progressive muscle relaxation, and exposure therapy can help, as well as therapeutic journaling or expressive writing.

Acceptance and Commitment Therapy

Acceptance and commitment therapy (ACT) is an approach that helps you accept/acknowledge your thoughts and feelings and identify the values important in your life so you can make adjustments to live in a way aligned with your values. Rather than trying to control or change your feelings and thoughts, it's about observing your feelings and thoughts without judgment or labeling emotions as "good" or "bad." Exercises and the use of metaphors help illustrate how you can gain awareness of your emotions and explore ways to change your relationship with your thoughts and feelings.

Addressing and Exploring Existential Concerns

Psychosocial oncology therapists are usually trained to approach and explore existential concerns, such as when patients want to address ways to live more meaningfully. Patients will often tell me—particularly after completing active treatment—that while they may have been happy before, they now want to focus more on what truly gives their lives meaning and purpose. It's fine if you *don't* feel this way, of course, but your cancer experience can provide a way for you to think about and review how you want to incorporate more meaning and purpose into your life.

Earlier in my career, I saw older patients, and very often those people in their seventies and eighties came to me with strong feelings of regret. They wished they had lived their lives differently, more aligned with what was important and meaningful to them. While we worked together on making changes in the present, oftentimes they still regretted not giving enough thought to their choices in the past. Such feelings are not nearly as common in young adults, who are normally so much more focused on reaching milestones that they don't often pause for this type of introspection.

One thing to consider: As much as my older patients regretted past life decisions, they rarely wished they had worked more. Even when their job was very aligned with their values, and gave their lives meaning, most still felt a lack of work-life balance. They regretted not spending more time connecting and sharing—with their families, the families they'd created among their friends, and in some cases their pets. You may not yet be in your golden years, but it's never too early to seek *your* best work-life balance, and consider those you most want to share it with.

Pause and Reflect

Some of my young adult cancer patients, however, feel that their diagnosis *does* give them a chance to pause, reflect, and—if the opportunity is there—make different life choices. If you think this might be you, try pondering these questions I often go through with them:

- What gives your life meaning?
- What gives your life purpose?
- How do you want to live?
- What are your priorities?
- What nourishes your spirit?
- What are you passionate about?
- When you look back in twenty, forty, or sixty years, how will you want your life to have gone?

You can still set goals if you decide to chart a new course, but you might want to think about them differently. Not just as objectives to *attain*, but as steps toward an even more meaningful and purposeful life. This approach centers around implementing meaning-focused life decisions and actions. Then, even if you feel emotionally overwhelmed, you can always go back and engage in those meaningful activities that give your life value.

Finding Meaning in Everyday Life

For some people, this may mean making different choices in the *type* of work that they do. Perhaps they are passionate about the environment, healthcare, or social justice, and so they may decide to switch to a field that is specifically tied to the mission or meaning that they want to bring to their life. Others may love what they do, and for them it is not so much about changing their careers as it is about finding different ways *outside* their jobs to live more meaningfully: volunteering, fundraising, or helping neighbors or family members facing their own challenges. Here are some potential outlets for meaningful living.

Spirituality and Religion

For many people, their faith is a critical part of how they view the world, find meaning, and cope with difficulties. Chaplains are employed by most hospitals and cancer centers, and they are usually nondenominational (with knowledge in many different religions). If you are already part of an organized religion, then staying connected to it—or reconnecting—can be very powerful. Prayer can be meditative and soothing for people who have that type of belief.

Participating in religious services also provides a sense of community support. I commonly hear from patients that members of their congregation have organized a "meal train" to drop meals off at their houses, or that congregants are taking turns driving them to chemotherapy.

Volunteering

Volunteering decreases feelings of sadness, loneliness, and anxiety. It can help you feel more connected to others and your values while doing something to make the world better. There are many volunteer opportunities out there—from holding babies in the ICU to working at an animal shelter to being a docent at a museum. The key is finding one that aligns with your beliefs; don't do something just because you think you "should."

There are a couple of concerns that I share with patients around volunteering. Just because you have/had cancer doesn't mean you need to volunteer working with cancer patients. If you decide to do so, however, I recommend waiting at least a year after completing your treatment before reaching out to others. Make sure to take care of yourself first.

Another thing to keep in mind when volunteering is to not overdo it. You don't need to make a huge time commitment to make a difference. If you are tremendously interested in the environment, for instance, you can go once a month to help clean up a beach. It should fit into your life, be doable, and provide a sense of fulfillment and internal reward.

Social Interactions

Social interactions and connections are an important part of a meaningful life and can contribute to your physical and mental health. We are social animals, but there is variability. Some people need or require more social contacts than others. Some people are energized by social interactions and some have a more limited social battery. Some enjoy big social gatherings, while others do not. Some prefer very intimate relationships, while others are not as interested or ready for that level of closeness, perhaps because they are still working out some aspects of their own lives. Some may prefer just brief daily social interactions, and then there are some who want it *all*—any type of connection, however brief or intimate, is fine by them. There is no correct way to find this type of fulfillment; it can come from whatever you find works best for you and meets your needs.

Psychopharmacology

As touched on earlier, psychopharmacology is a specialty field within psychiatry focused on the study and use of medications used in treating mental disorders. The goal when dealing with cancer treatment is to do everything you can to help yourself through the experience. If psychiatric medication is part of that equation, this will require your being under the care of a psychiatrist who can write prescriptions. It is preferable the psychiatrist understands how your cancer treatment, medications, and medical changes can impact your mental health; is familiar with drug interactions; and is well versed in addressing cancer-related pain as part of a team.

In some cases it could be physical pain related to treatment—such as terrible headaches or gastrointestinal issues—causing your depression or anxiety. Psychiatrists trained in psychosocial oncology understand it is important to treat the pain while still addressing the mood changes. Perhaps after treating your pain, your mood improves. They know the side effects that cancer treatments can cause and the right (and safe) medications for dealing with them. For example, there are medications to help with concentration due to chemo brain, and being trained in this area helps psychiatrists recognize the specific ways to intervene. Since it is not always easy to find a psychiatrist trained in psychosocial oncology, you might first want to get a consultation with one, and then they can make suggestions to your oncology team or your primary physician on how to follow up and prescribe.

Key Points

- Many young cancer patients can benefit from talking to a professional about their experience at some point during (and after) their journey.
- It's best to find a mental health provider who is specially trained in working with early onset cancer patients. They will understand the effects of treatment and what is happening to your body, including the impact of different medications on your physical and emotional well-being.

- Group therapy is a great way to address the social isolation that you might be facing. There are many different types of groups (in person and virtual), so explore and try to find one that works for you.
- Professionals can also help you explore specific therapies, such as CBT and ACT, that could help you manage your mental health.

CHAPTER 8
Post-Treatment Life

For Brook, who identifies as nonbinary (using "they/them" as their preferred pronouns), college provided an opportunity to explore their sense of self through a great group of friends—including a girlfriend. So after being diagnosed with lymphoma their junior year, and forced to take a semester off for treatment, Brook, twenty-one, chose to go to a cancer center near school rather than return to their family's home out of state.

"Things were tense with my family since I came out a couple years before," Brook recalls. "They had a hard time accepting me, and I felt like my friends would be more supportive as I went through chemo therapy."

Their parents did surprise Brook by coming to town to help out during their active treatment, but they quickly returned home once it was done. Brook's hair had all come back, along with their weight, so their parents assumed everything was fine. So did Brook.

"Unfortunately, I did not expect things would still be so tough after treatment," says Brook. "When I told my girlfriend how much I missed seeing my oncology team every couple weeks, and was worried about my cancer coming back, she didn't get it. She just couldn't deal with my emotions, so we broke up."

Returning to school was also a challenge. Brook now tired easily, sometimes falling asleep in class, and struggled to keep up. Friends who figured Brook would be "back to normal" couldn't understand why they didn't like going to parties anymore. After getting through cancer, didn't they appreciate life more than ever?

"I figured that would be the case too, but I just felt exhausted and overwhelmed by everything," explains Brook. "I went to a cancer psychologist, who recommended I talk to my professors about accommodations. They offered me extra time on tests, but it was all the assignments and deadlines outside class that were stressing me the most. The psychologist told me I had something called 'chemo brain,' and even wrote a letter to my academic advisor explaining what that meant."

Eventually, with help from therapy, Brook learned to be more patient with their recovery and use strategies to not agonize so much about a possible recurrence. They gradually regained their energy, caught up in school, and started going out socially again. By accepting some things would never be quite the same, they also came to believe that life after treatment—their "new normal"—could still be satisfying.

Now What?

The end of cancer treatment is not always quite what you expect. I often hear comments like these from patients:

- "Everyone in my family just wants things to go back to normal, but it's different for me now."
- "I don't know who I am. I feel so lost."
- "I still worry about every lump or pain. In the days leading up to my scans, my anxiety is off the charts."

This chapter is going to focus on some of the changes and concerns you may encounter at the end of your treatment. Hopefully you're going to be around for many more years, so there is a lot to focus on. What's most important to remember is that it's not only about surviving, it's also about *how* you survive—as some patients say, "it's not just surviving; it's about thriving."

Until very recently, most of the concentration on how people handle the completion of cancer treatment centered on children and older adults rather than those ages eighteen to forty-nine. In the years before search engines and social media profiles made us all much easier to track down, it was often difficult to follow up with young adult cancer survivors. They might have changed jobs numerous times since their treatment and/or moved to different cities, states, and even countries from where they received care. In addition, many of them who were on their parents' insurance when they started treatment in their late teens or twenties had later switched to their own insurance and transferred their records to parts unknown. In recent years, thanks to electronic medical records and other ways to stay in touch, there is increased attention to follow-up care for patients in this stage in life.

More Change (and More Uncertainty)

I can attest from working with young adults post-treatment that as a group, they tend to have very mixed feelings about completing treatment. While they are certainly happy and relieved to be leaving blood draws and infusions behind, many of them—including Brook, the patient quoted at the start of this chapter—are also nervous, sad, and unsure of the future. This jumble of emotions is not what they expected, and it surprises them. Perhaps you've experienced these feelings too.

One reason may be the abruptness of it all. After you finish treatment, everyone makes a big deal and celebrates. Then your oncology team basically says, "Go live your life, and we'll see you in three months." You've spent months, sometimes even *years*, coming to the cancer center on a regular basis. Your doctors, nurses, and other clinicians have essentially become part of your extended family. Now they are telling you that they'll see you in three months. That sudden decrease in access to your oncology team—and its support—can be difficult. You may feel a sense of being unmoored, or even abandoned. While you know that coming in less often is a *good* thing, you might not be prepared for these feelings.

If this is the case, you are not alone. Research studies show young adults completing cancer treatment report needing more support and more information and often feeling more disoriented than expected. They often feel ill prepared to move forward, wondering things like, "How do I go on with my life? Who am I now? How do I get back to normal?"

Facing a New Fear

This period is when many patients are referred to me for the first time. Upon our meeting, they will often describe trying to address feelings that they have put on hold while dealing with treatment, and finding that they are not sure how to deal with them or quite ready to do so at this time.

One thing I hear a lot is that while they certainly didn't like being in treatment, they felt a sense of security knowing that at least they were doing *something* to fight their cancer—or, in some cases, prevent it from returning. Like Brook, they are no longer taking action with chemo or radiation, and so they start to worry more about the cancer coming back.

Fear of Cancer Recurrence

Fear of cancer recurrence (FCR) is defined as a fear, worry, or concern regarding the possibility that one's cancer will return, progress, or metastasize. FCR is quite common, with studies showing anywhere from 31 percent to 82 percent of cancer patients reporting it. In the case of young adults, who expect to live many more years post-treatment than older survivors, the uneasiness often extends to fears of developing a new cancer in the future.

Young adults with children are at an even higher risk for clinically significant FCR than their peers without kids. So are those individuals with high levels of anxiety or symptoms of post-traumatic stress—such as flashbacks of their treatment—who tend to avoid situations that remind them of it. One particularly challenging form of FCR at all ages is "scanxiety," which describes the specific type of anxiety you feel both before getting scans and while waiting for their results.

In managing FCR, the first thing to acknowledge is that these feelings are normal. Everybody who has been through cancer is going to experience FCR to some degree, especially around anniversaries such as the date you were diagnosed, the date you started chemo, and the date you finished treatment. It's also quite common to have FCR in the days just before follow-up visits and while waiting for the results of scans, blood work, or other tests. Additional triggers can come when someone you know has a recurrence, and you get to wondering if you're next, or if you hear that a young adult celebrity has been diagnosed with cancer.

For most people, anxiety and fear around a recurrence will gradually improve over time. Cancer will not always be the center of your life, but it will never totally go away either. It may recede into the background as you get further away from the end of your active treatment, yet still be somewhere in the back of your mind. There might be times, even years later, when it will reemerge to the surface—especially on follow-up visits. That's expected, as long as you don't let your FCR disrupt you to the point where you stop taking care of yourself or the fear interferes with your functioning.

Ways to Manage FCR

Remember—every new physical symptom doesn't mean cancer. It is important for you to decipher the possible cause(s) of a new physical symptom before immediately assuming that it is a recurrence or new cancer.

Let's say, for instance, that every time you start to feel abdominal pain or cold-like symptoms post-treatment, your first thought is, "Oh no, has the cancer come back?" This may be understandable, but unless the pain is sudden and severe and you require emergency help, you could try to take a step back and analyze the situation. Maybe your abdominal pain can be attributed to something other than cancer. Try asking yourself questions like these (which can be tweaked accordingly to fit other post-treatment issues):

- Did I participate in an exercise that could have resulted in my abdominal discomfort?
- Did I pull a muscle?
- Did I eat something that could have caused my GI distress?

- Is there a GI virus or bug going around? Could I have caught this from someone?
- Am I congested or feeling run-down because I've pushed myself too much, or might it be due to allergies?
- Could I be more fatigued than usual, as well as congested, because I've been around somebody who has/had a cold?
- When did my symptoms start? Are they worsening or improving over time?
- Is there anything I can do to lessen the discomfort?

Asking these questions should go a long way toward helping you analyze your symptoms more objectively. Of course, if at any point your symptoms become too much to handle physically and/or are causing you excessive anxiety, it's best to call your oncology team and/or go to the ER. There is no need to wait and suffer.

Following are further suggestions that can help you manage FCR:

- **Learn to recognize your own FCR and anxiety triggers.** Common triggers we discussed earlier include anniversary dates, learning someone you know has had a recurrence, or waiting for test results, but try to identify what other specific things prompt your fears. Maybe it's a particular physical symptom, or a certain place, that serves as the instigator. If you can determine what (and where) serves as your triggers, you can find ways to avoid those situations—or, if avoiding is not helpful, then at least better prepare for them.
- **Rather than catastrophizing (jumping to the worst possible conclusions), try and reframe your thoughts and feelings around FCR.** Make an effort to allow and acknowledge your thoughts and feelings by pulling back and really examining them for what they are: words you've constructed in your mind. Visualize them as being written on a chalkboard or up in neon lights. Rather than becoming one with your thoughts and feelings, try to detach and become an *observer* of them.

- **Work with your oncology team to schedule follow-up appointments as soon as possible after scans, blood work, or other tests.** This way you need not wait too many long, excruciating days for results, or risk seeing them on your electronic medical record before having a chance to discuss them with your team.

- **Develop a routine to help yourself feel better on scan and test days.** Consider wearing a lucky shirt that you associate with good results, or take a walk outside between appointments to get some fresh air.

- **Plan ahead to end scan and test days—regardless of the outcome—with a special treat, such as visiting a museum or a favorite café or restaurant.** This will give you something to look forward to after each follow-up appointment. Also, if you are working, plan to take the entire day off. Even if your appointment doesn't seem like it will take very long—and even if all the results are good—you may need the whole day to deal with any emotions stemming from the experience.

- **Lower your stress level and regulate your emotions by practicing mindfulness meditation (or other meditation).** There are many wonderful forms of meditation to help manage your anxiety and FCR, including apps you can access on your phone or tablet. It might be especially helpful to practice your meditation of choice in the days leading up to tests, or while waiting for test results from your oncology team, but you can really use it anytime you feel FCR coming on.

- **Engage in physical exercise or movement, whether on your own, with a friend or partner, or as part of a group or team.** Anything from walking to more intense workouts can do wonders for your mood, and help take your mind—at least temporarily—off your fears.

All these ideas hearken back to the concept of fight-or-flight (discussed in Chapter 2)—and how you react when you are about to encounter something potentially life-threatening. Since the results of scans, blood work, and other tests *could* be a threat to both your life and well-being, logic dictates that it is normal and expected for you to feel anxiety in the days approaching follow-up visits. However, if anxiety and fear of recurrence continue to interfere with your quality of life for days or weeks leading up to these visits, you may benefit from a consult with a mental health professional.

Adjusting to Your New Normal

Many young adults—and cancer patients of *all* ages—expect that within a week or two of finishing active treatment, they will feel fine and return to their old, pre-cancer life. In my experience, this is not the case. As I often tell my patients, how can you expect to recover so quickly after being in treatment for six months, a year, or even longer? Just as it takes time for your hair to grow back after falling out, the inside of your body needs to recover.

This period, starting with the end of treatment and continuing well into post-treatment, is what I often refer to as "finding your new normal." It is a time for reexamining who you are now that you have gone through cancer. Often patients will tell me that they just want to "go back to normal" after treatment. What they mean is the *old* normal, before they *started* treatment. But taking that approach, I acknowledge, may be challenging. Here is a how I explain it:

Normal → Cancer → New Normal*
* *Your new normal = your old normal + your cancer experience.*

The point is this: Cancer cannot simply be erased from your lived experience. *It happened.* Much of the work I do is to help young adults work through and integrate their old selves—who they were—into who they are now due to the emotional, physical, cognitive, and spiritual changes they've experienced. This often means exploring feelings set aside during treatment and having an opportunity to process and make sense of them.

Avoid Comparisons to Your Old Life

One thing I suggest is to try *not* to compare yourself—especially physically—to who you were before. Gradually, over months, you will notice your energy coming back. Emphasize this as a positive, rather than focusing how you still lack your pre-cancer stamina. That's your *old* normal. In terms of your recovery, it is best to compare how you feel *today* with how you felt at the very end of treatment. Remember, it's like your hair growing back. It's a step-by-step process that takes time.

I understand that's easier said than done. Patience is a hard concept to grasp when you're young and used to bouncing back quickly from challenges. Your inclination is to just plow ahead, but you need to keep in mind that cancer is different than anything you've dealt with before. Your body has endured a lot, physically and emotionally. Patients sometimes describe experiencing an inner battle with themselves in which they set up unrealistic expectations for their recovery and then become frustrated when they fail to meet them.

If you've done this as well, that's okay. It's a natural response to the situation, because you likely already feel you've missed out on so much during your treatment. Depending on your age, you may believe you have fallen behind your peers in school or at work, or missed out on other important life events. If you have kids, you've probably been unable to attend some games, recitals, and other events. It's natural to want to jump back into life as quickly as possible.

Patient Voices

"My treatment ending and my new normal starting was blurry. While I was excited and ready to start life again, it was a slow and frustrating process. I was not suddenly better; rather, I was now adjusting to a new chronic illness, a lifetime of medications and appointments, and a new awareness of my mortality that my peers couldn't relate to. I didn't let it stop me, though. I found a good mental health provider, began physical therapy, and started to build back a life that feels fulfilling." —Ashlyn H.

What it all comes down to is learning to accept your new normal. Try not to measure yourself against your peers. You may lament what you might have missed out on, but try also to embrace each new day and plan future adventures. Focus on yourself and your own recovery. While it's going to have its ups and downs, the important thing is you are still here. You've already proven you can get through cancer, and you can get through this period too.

I will often see young adult cancer survivors for individual therapy sessions for a year or more as they work through their recovery and find their "new normal." In some cases, patients will return to see me much later on when dealing with a "new normal" change such as becoming parents through fertility treatment or adoption. To them, and all my patients, I emphasize this: *Your new normal is ever evolving, and ever changing, throughout your life.*

Practice Self-Compassion

One of the main ways that I work with patients to help them deal with post-treatment issues and lingering side effects is by guiding them into practicing self-compassion. This entails being patient with yourself, recognizing all you've been through in terms of your treatment—its impact on your body as well as your emotions—and then giving yourself time to heal. We all talk to ourselves; try using self-compassion and talking to yourself in a kind voice. If you're having trouble envisioning how this works, ask yourself these questions:

- If it were somebody else who had just endured what you did, how would you tell them to act toward themselves?
- If you could watch your life as a movie, how would you view yourself and your experiences so far?

Now take those answers and try to direct them at yourself. Watch out for your critical inner voice, and engage in self-talk with caring and understanding.

Don't be discouraged if this seems really hard; it is for lots of people. You might be very kind and compassionate toward others, but when it comes to *your own* well-being, that's a different story. You may set unrealistic expectations for your recovery and drive yourself too hard to reach them. Self-compassion means realizing that the end of treatment doesn't mean that everything will go back to the way it was. That version of you may no longer exist in the same way as before, but your new normal can still be very fulfilling.

Post-Treatment Side Effects

As you establish your new normal, you'll quickly learn that you're not immediately free of side effects just because your treatment has officially ended. There are many different potential *post-treatment* side effects to contend with depending on your type and stage of cancer as well as your course of treatment. We won't try to describe them all. Along with fatigue and chemo brain, here are some of the bigger general concerns I hear from patients:

- **Weight changes:** Some people gain weight, and some people lose it. Either way, try not to get discouraged. The nutrition recommendations during treatment are often different than they are post-treatment, so seek the advice of a registered dietitian with a specialty in oncology survivorship and post-treatment health. They can help you develop a diet that works within your lifestyle, including new foods you might want to consider, as well as provide pointers on how to make sure you always get enough fluids—hydration being central to any healthy diet.
- **Muscles and muscle mass:** This can especially be an issue for people who were very active prior to their diagnosis. During treatment, you likely did a lot more sitting and sleeping than normal, so now you need to work your way back muscle-wise. Enlisting the assistance of a physical therapist or exercise physiologist with oncology expertise can help you set realistic

expectations for yourself. Making the appointment for an initial fitness evaluation is the first step and is homework I often give to my patients. Programs like Livestrong (at some YMCAs) are specifically designed to help cancer survivors regain their strength.

- **Body image:** Depending on how your body was affected by the cancer, you might look different or have things you can no longer do the way you could before. This can also influence how you feel about yourself. If you had an osteosarcoma, for instance, you may have scars or have lost part or all of a limb or limbs. It takes time to adjust to such changes. Be patient and kind with yourself. Remember that there is more assistance than ever for people with physical impairments or disabilities. If you need inspiration, and a peek at what you *can* do, check out the stories of Jamie Whitmore and Mark Barr, young adult cancer survivors who went on to compete in the Paralympics.

Post-Treatment Cancer-Related Fatigue

While it would be logical to assume that, as a young adult, your energy would quickly return once your treatment ended, that is unfortunately not usually the case. No matter how strong you are, or *think* you are, cancer is tough to bounce back from. Young adults are unprepared for this circumstance, and are confused by it.

Cancer-related fatigue, both during and after treatment, has been found in some studies to be more prevalent and of higher severity among young adults. Studies designed to assess CRF have shown that patients ages forty-nine and younger reported fatigue more often than those age fifty and above. Perhaps this has to do with all the demands you're typically dealing with during this time of life—from school to careers to caregiving. Once treatment is over, you and everyone around you expects that you'll pick up where you left off prior to diagnosis. That's a stressful expectation in itself.

Other factors can also lead to post-treatment CRF, such as struggling with body image concerns, financial and insurance worries, and being on endocrine treatment for breast cancer. Ongoing anxiety, depression, emotional distress, pain, sleep difficulties, menopausal symptoms, and medical comorbidities are possible contributors to CRF as well.

Post-treatment CRF usually improves gradually, over time, but it can take anywhere from six months to a year—and sometimes even longer—before you will truly feel energetic again. CRF is multidimensional: It has a physical component, an emotional component, a cognitive component, and a spiritual component. It is also distressing, persistent, and subjective. Part of what makes it so difficult to manage is that it *is* so subjective—and not easily quantifiable. Doctors do not know the exact cause(s) of post-treatment CRF. You can't get a scan that shows the cause or degree of your fatigue. You can *feel* it, but you can't measure it.

Energy consumption is not always easy for us—or others—to measure either. Here is an example I give in explaining post-treatment CRF to new patients: While it is clear how and why one might be exhausted after completing an eight- or ten-hour shift at a physical job like landscaping or construction, it is *not* so clear as to how somebody who sits all day could feel similarly wiped out after eight or ten hours. Believe me, they can. After sitting all day talking with people, I feel cognitively and emotionally tired. Even without lifting heavy barbells or bricks, you can exert plenty of cognitive, emotional, and spiritual energy on various meetings or projects.

To help address post-treatment CRF, I suggest that patients first examine how they are currently using their precious energy and then make changes accordingly, pacing themselves to fit their circumstances. This practice can work for you too. If you are putting a lot of energy into a cognitive task—such as problem-solving, for instance—you may find you have less left to tackle something physical that same day. Think of your energy during this period as a finite resource. Consider your agenda for any given day, and then allot your energy accordingly. Keep in mind that putting it toward one thing will mean less energy for something else—you can't continually add more tasks to your plate. You only have so much strength to give.

It's very helpful to pace and to plan, even if it feels odd at first. One key suggestion you may remember from our chapters on active treatment is that if you know you're doing something special at day's end—maybe going out to dinner and/or to a movie—you should try and find ways to take it easier in the hours beforehand. While such preparation may on the surface seem unnecessary for somebody young and done with active treatment, it can do wonders.

Here are a few more suggestions for dealing with post-treatment CRF:

- **Learn the difference between when you're feeling tired versus totally exhausted.** Once you find where that point exists for yourself, you can hopefully learn to listen to your body—and not push yourself so much that you wind up out of commission for several days.
- **Exercise and move.** While counterintuitive, it does work: Exercising is one of the best ways to improve your energy. The longer you *don't* move, the more fatigued you will feel. The key is to gradually increase your activity post-treatment, not overdo it, and not work out too close to your bedtime.
- **Consider CBT.** CBT (cognitive behavioral therapy—described in Chapter 7) is a combination of psycho-education and specific strategies to target distinct symptoms or behavior, including fatigue. For example, CBT strategies could help you learn to identify the difference between tired and exhausted.
- **Don't assume sleep will fix the problem.** While getting some long- or short-term shut-eye is vital at certain points in your cancer treatment cycle, it does not guarantee you will wake up refreshed when dealing with post-treatment CRF. If you are struggling with chronic sleeplessness, cognitive behavioral therapy for insomnia (CBT-I) may help.
- **Check your meds.** A medical-management review by your oncology team will determine any underlying causes of fatigue related to your current medications. Use this opportunity to

discuss pharmacological interventions for fatigue with your oncology team, such as the short-term use of a drug like modafinil.

- **Check your blood counts for possible anemia.** Fatigue is one of the main symptoms of anemia.
- **Try integrative therapies.** These modalities, such as acupuncture and meditation, can be very helpful in tackling stress.

Note that what usually works best is a combination of these options. In the end, it all goes back to the same concept I've passed on before: You need to accept that you just can't keep going, going, going as in the past. You won't have that endless energy you are accustomed to drawing on, so it's important to prioritize, pace, and, more than anything, remind yourself to be patient and self-compassionate. This is one of the hardest things for most young people post-treatment, because they expect everything will immediately go back to the way it was. But try to remember, that was the *old* normal—and you are now adjusting to your evolving and ever-changing *new* normal. Your stamina will gradually improve, but it takes time.

Post-Treatment Chemo Brain

You may remember our discussion of CRCI (cancer-related cognitive impairment), also known as chemo brain, from the earlier chapters on active treatment. CRCI can include difficulties with attention, memory, concentration, language (word finding), processing speed, and executive function related to cancer treatment. Multitasking becomes more difficult when dealing with chemo brain, as does planning ahead and anticipating problems. Your ability to process information, concentrate, and pay attention to detail is temporarily diminished, and that can cause performance problems at school or work. Differences in your cognitive functioning, however subtle, can still have a big impact on your *overall* functioning.

Like CRF, CRCI can persist into post-treatment. And while things do improve over time, this initial period can be a challenge if you assume you will immediately be able to function cognitively as you did before treatment. We don't know the exact reason(s) for chemo brain, although there are likely multiple causes. If the specific cancer you had affects the central nervous system, and you received chemotherapy or radiation to this area, that is likely a contributing factor. If you did *not* have cancer of the central nervous system, here are some other possible contributing factors to chemo brain:

- Type and dose of chemotherapy
- Adjunct cancer treatments (like endocrine therapy or immunotherapy)
- Patient demographics (age, gender, etc.)
- Other medical conditions (such as diabetes)
- Preexisting ADHD or ADD
- Medications that can affect concentration, such as steroids or thyroid medications
- Anxiety and/or depression
- Premature menopause due to treatment
- Fatigue and/or difficulties sleeping

There are quite a few ways to try to circumvent the challenges presented by CRCI. These include:

- **Practicing self-compassion:** As stated earlier, this is a great way to deal with cancer-related fatigue and other post-treatment side effects. It can help with CRCI too. Remind yourself of everything that you and your body have been through, and that recovery takes time.
- **Getting moving:** Any type of exercise is good for your overall health, of course, but it can also help manage issues like anxiety and depression that may contribute to CRCI.
- **Managing your stress:** Anxiety interferes with your ability to assimilate and process information. Finding ways to destress, either on a regular, structured basis or in moments you feel

yourself getting too anxious, can be extremely beneficial. We've discussed many methods in previous chapters; whatever worked for you during treatment—mindfulness meditation, prayer, yoga, music therapy, etc.—may help you at this point as well.

- **Inquiring about medications:** Speak with your team about meds that can help improve your attention and concentration, such as short-term use of psychostimulants.
- **Going for testing:** Neuropsychological testing with a psychologist who's knowledgeable about the effects of cancer treatment on cognitive functioning can be very helpful.
- **Using software:** Neuropsychologists may suggest you try computerized cognitive-training programs to help with improving your memory and concentration.
- **Consulting with an expert:** Try educational and vocational counseling.
- **Considering CBT, integrative therapy, and/or medication management and intervention:** These strategies can all be very helpful, and a combination of approaches often works best.

Reestablishing Friendships

In addition to reassessing your physical and mental health as your treatment ends and your "new normal" begins, you will also likely find that your relationships with friends and loved ones have changed. You might even hear comments that can add to your feelings of frustration, such as:

- "You are so lucky that it was caught early."
- "But you're cured—why aren't you happy? What more could you want?"
- "It's over. Now you can forget all about it and go back to the way you were."

Remember the concept of toxic positivity we discussed in Chapter 5—those well-intentioned but misguided things people often say after you're diagnosed? Just like those statements, these show an ignorance to what you're going through, only now it's related to post-treatment. This section will offer some guidance on navigating the tricky situations you could encounter with people around you.

You may find that once you begin relinquishing any dependence on your caregivers and venturing back out on your own, the friendships you enjoyed prior to or during your cancer journey are no longer quite the same.

Patient Voices

"Being a young adult with cancer is paradoxical. We are taught that one is either young and healthy or old and sick. Upon my diagnosis of cancer at age twenty-one, I found myself at the intersection of youth and illness—I now occupy multiple conflicting identities. The disease is an erratic bulldozer. However, through my young adult cancer advocacy, my graduate studies, and a newfound vulnerability and depth within my friendships, I have reconstructed my sense of self and notion of success."
—Sarah D.

Dealing with Cancer Ghosting

While many friends and family may have been extremely supportive during each stage of your treatment, others might *not* have been there for you—a situation that can leave you with unresolved feelings post-treatment. In some cases, it has been the people that you least expected who have shined the brightest, and those you *most* expected to step up who have stayed distant. Now, as you go about reestablishing yourself in the world, you may not know quite what to do about these relationships.

The word "ghosting" has emerged in recent years to describe the act of suddenly and inexplicably breaking off all communication with another person. Cancer ghosting can emerge when you share your diagnosis with friends and then stop hearing from them. No calls. No texts. No contact of any kind, even when you try and initiate a virtual conversation and can see that they have viewed your message. Some recipients of cancer ghosting say it can be harder to handle than treatment, because at least they can understand *why* they feel crappy during chemo.

What could cause someone to desert you during such a challenging time in your life? We have already touched in earlier chapters on the fact that because of your age, fewer of your peers have an understanding of what it's like to go through a major illness like cancer. Accordingly, someone who can't grasp what you are experiencing may be unsure when or how to reach out. They might even be afraid to do so, a sort of fear of the unknown—or of saying the wrong thing.

While this doesn't justify the lack of even a *Hello, how have you been?* text, it should give you some solace that their behavior is not indicative of any shortcomings on *your* part. You may, in fact, never know the real reason. Each relationship is different, and how you choose to respond—or not respond—is a very individual decision. Coming to grips with feelings of loss, sadness, and anger about how these people behaved, and learning how to deal with these emotions, is a major focus of discussion for many of the young adults that I see.

You might have some of the same emotions. There may be people who have long been in your life, and have supported you before, but just couldn't "deal" with your cancer. How do you integrate what's happened to the relationship? There's no right answer to that, but what's important is accepting the situation with as little judgment as possible—and then choosing the most comfortable path forward.

Sharing Your Recovery Reality

Another challenge you might encounter is how to communicate to your friends that even though it's been three months (or six months, or one year) since your treatment ended, you are not yet able to be as active as they—or you—would like. Even if you *look* better, you just might not have the energy to pick up where you left off. Sometimes people get it, and sometimes they don't. All you can do is explain things to them in a way they can hopefully understand . . . and if they *can't*, what does that mean in terms of the relationship?

To deal with these issues and ambiguities, try to find a way to bring your family and friends up to speed as soon as possible post-treatment. Share not only what you're still going through, but also what they should *expect* from you. Help prepare others for your recovery at the same time you are preparing yourself. Remember some of the unrealistic expectations you may have had at the end of treatment? Chances are, your family and friends are in the same boat. If you thought, for instance, that you'd be back to your "old normal" within a month, you can be sure they will think that as well.

If you want to cut down on their unthinking comments, you need to help prepare your loved ones for what lies ahead. Make them part of the same education that you go through. Have them join you for counseling, or share books, articles, and videos focused on post-treatment challenges. As you form and design your own recovery timeline, make sure they know it as well. The more you are all on the same page, the better.

Just as it's important to talk openly about your goals, feelings, and fears with your friends and family, you should encourage them to do the same. If they have questions or concerns, it's better that you know about them. The best scenario is to find a balance, so that everyone feels they can share their thoughts in a beneficial but not detrimental way. Just like you have to remind yourself to be patient with yourself, you will likely need to remind your family and friends that recovery is slow. Remember, this is a whole new experience for *all of you*.

Addressing Survivor's Guilt

Another concern I hear a lot from patients involves the strong, persistent feelings of sadness and remorse they experience, often post-treatment, around their being alive while other cancer patients they know have experienced a relapse or recurrence or died. These emotions can be confusing and intrusive, because they are likely coming just as you and those close to you are trying to celebrate your milestone.

This experience is called "survivor's guilt." You've made it to this point in your cancer journey, which is certainly *worth* acknowledging positively, but others you may have met during your treatment or at other points in your life were not so fortunate. It is only natural, therefore, to be left wondering things like:

- "Why did I survive, when this other person I sat next to in chemo didn't?"
- "Why did I not experience as many side effects as my friend who was on the exact same treatment?"
- "Why can I still have kids after treatment, and others can't?"

First, be assured that your feelings are completely normal—survivor's guilt is more prevalent than you might think. Consider the interviews you hear after a natural disaster or mass shooting, when people tell reporters that they can't believe they made it through while others did not. These widely different emotions can coexist for you as well: You can be both grateful for your own situation *and* simultaneously sad or even angry about what others had to endure. As we have discussed before, we can experience two or more contrasting emotions at the same time. It is not an either/or situation.

Survivor's guilt is not necessarily easy to manage, especially when loved ones minimize such feelings with placating comments like, "Just be happy you're okay." While you can feel a sense of helplessness, anger, or injustice that other deserving patients did not survive, you must accept that there is unfortunately no "justice" when it comes to cancer. And as difficult as it may be, it is also important to try and not let this guilt fester. Do your best to address these emotions early on to avoid other possible problems with your mood, sleep habits, and concentration. Practice self-compassion, and remind yourself that these feelings *are* normal.

It takes time to grieve, just as it takes time to heal. How you deal with these losses is for *you* to decide. Like so many things we are talking about in this book, there is no one strategy that works for everyone in terms of honoring a person. You could decide to plant a tree, attend an end-of-life event, or take part in a cancer fundraising walk. You could also honor someone's memory by taking steps to make things better for others down the road, such as volunteering or getting involved in cancer advocacy. Often seemingly small gestures can be the most meaningful, and also help you most in coping with the loss, such as looking at pictures of you with the person or expressing your emotions through painting or photography—using positive thoughts about a lost friend as artistic inspiration.

In-person or online support groups can also be a great resource to help guide you on this path. Some groups, in fact, are geared specifically toward young adults coping with post-treatment, and survivor's guilt often comes up during discussions. By talking with and hearing from others in your situation, and acknowledging what you are feeling, you will likely experience a sense of validation. You may also learn ways others are coping with their survivor's guilt.

Key Points

- The end of your treatment does not mean an end to side effects, fatigue, and emotional ups and downs. You can address those physical and mental health symptoms with similar self-care techniques to those you used during treatment, such as exercise, hydration, and therapy.
- Your life post-treatment is *not* the same as your life pre-diagnosis—it simply can't be. It can still, however, be fulfilling and happy.
- Practice self-compassion as you gauge your energy levels post-treatment, and set realistic expectations both for yourself and others around your daily capabilities.
- Cancer-related fatigue can still be an issue post-treatment, as can chemo brain. While both may persist for quite some time, several possible interventions can lessen their impact.
- Survivor's guilt is a common response when you make it through treatment but know others who did not. Try to honor their lives even as you continue living yours.

CHAPTER 9
Sexual Health

The changes came when Chloe least expected them. She would be at work, going about her business, and then suddenly begin sweating profusely despite the air conditioner humming behind her. At lunch a friend would stop her mid-sentence, asking with concern why Chloe looked all bright red and flustered. Even at night, with her open bedroom window letting in the cool breeze, she would awaken at all hours—her sheets drenched in sweat.

What Chloe was experiencing were hot flashes, a common sign of menopause caused by hormonal changes. But unlike most women, who go through this change of life naturally in their late forties to early fifties, she was dealing with it at age twenty-six. Chloe had recently completed treatment for hormone-receptor-positive (HR+) breast cancer, including a mastectomy, chemotherapy, and reconstruction. She was now taking monthly injections of the drug Lupron, along with hormone therapy, as part of her oncology team's efforts to prevent a recurrence by lowering her estrogen levels. The approach, Chloe's doctor explained, would also put her into "temporary premature menopause."

"None of my friends in their twenties could understand what I was going through, and I was too uncomfortable and embarrassed to try and explain," recalls Chloe. "Then, in addition to the hot flashes, I started getting more easily irritated and emotional. It was like being premenstrual all the time."

Chloe's problems extended into her romantic life. She had less interest in sex with her boyfriend, and when their intimacy included sexual intercourse, the vaginal pain was extreme. She had thought she was willing to do anything to keep the cancer from coming back, but now she wasn't so sure.

"When I finally told my oncologist how much the treatment was bothering me, she recommended I talk to a psychologist on the sexual health team at the cancer center," says Chloe. "I didn't think therapy could help with issues like these, but it wasn't just talking. It was focused on specific steps that could make a big difference."

After reassuring Chloe that both her hot flashes and sex-related issues—which included vaginal dryness and reduced elasticity—were common and treatable, the psychologist made recommendations to her oncology team. Chloe was prescribed sessions of pelvic floor physical therapy, which taught her how to relax her vaginal muscles for more comfortable intercourse, and she was given a vaginal moisturizer to help with dryness. The hot flashes, irritability, and restless nights improved with her being prescribed citalopram.

"The psychologist also encouraged me to get a vibrator, and start experimenting by myself and with my boyfriend to find what felt comfortable sexually post-cancer," explains Chloe. "I thought it would be really awkward, but it actually brought us closer together."

What Nobody Talks About

When I started my clinical practice more than thirty years ago, young adults would be referred to me during their cancer treatment. As I started going through my regular intake with them, I would ask if they had noticed any changes in their sexual life. I knew that depression or severe anxiety could bring about changes in sexual desire—usually *less* desire—so that was partly why I asked. What surprised me was how often I would get answers like this:

"Yes, I have less sexual desire, and I'm so concerned that I'm beginning to wonder if it is going to be like this for the rest of my life."

The problem was that these patients had been completely blindsided by the situation. Nobody had explained or even mentioned to them that a change in their sexual life, often less sexual desire, could happen as a side effect of cancer treatment. Many of them were indeed anxious or depressed, in part *because* of the change in their sexual functioning. It was impacting their sense of well-being across the board, just like the cancer was.

I still remember one patient who was very upset about his situation. He was young and single, and a major part of his sense of identity was dating. Now, however, he had little to no interest in sex. He tried to masturbate, seeking to spark some desire—visually, by looking at movies, anything he could think of—but that didn't help either. It was a total change. He asked me if it was always going to be like this, and I told him that based on his diagnosis and treatment, his sexual desire would probably return six months to a year post-treatment. If it did not come back by then, I added, he should let me know.

That young man never returned to see me, but about a year and a half later, I saw him in the cancer center lobby. He noticed me and, without saying anything, gave me a thumbs-up. I took that to mean things had returned to normal. I was glad for his happy result, but I realized in dealing with so many similar cases that I had very limited knowledge on sexual health during and after cancer treatment. All I could provide was psycho-education based on my clinical experience. So I took it upon myself to get training, which enabled me to begin practicing sexual health therapy with cancer patients.

The good news is that we've gotten a lot better since the 1990s at understanding this issue. However, it remains my clinical experience—and research confirms this—that sexual health is *still* not addressed enough as part of cancer care. When you're first diagnosed, this makes sense; you're fearful for your future, and your focus is naturally going to be on the cancer. Sex is not on your mind, nor your oncologist's. Everything is geared toward devising the best possible treatment plan.

But we know through studies of young adult patients that if their healthcare professionals do not bring it up, they do not inquire—even though they report desiring more information about the impact their cancer diagnoses and treatments have on sex. So while we *are* better today at bringing up fertility issues and treatment options to patients, it's clear their cancer-related sexual concerns are not focused on enough at the start or any other point of treatment. This is especially the case for LGBTQ+ patients. It is important, therefore, that you advocate for yourself and ask for information rather than wait for it—even if you feel awkward doing so. This chapter will provide a very general overview of sexual health and give you suggestions of some questions that you may want to ask your medical team.

It is important to note that when I see patients for therapy related to sexual health, I first do so individually. Then, if they have a partner or partners, I later bring them in if necessary. The information provided here is going to be very general; there is no way that I could cover all the different types of cancer and the various ways they can impact your sexual life. There is also no way to include all the variables that affect us as sexual beings. Still, this broad overview will provide a foundation to explore what sexual health looks like for you during cancer treatment and beyond.

Factors That Affect Sexual Health During Treatment

Many young adults undergoing cancer treatment will experience some change in their sexual lives. I feel this topic is so important that it should be discussed along with other possible side effects. So when your doctor tells you that you may lose your hair or experience nausea and/or fatigue, they should also mention that you could experience changes in your sexual life and your sexual functioning—usually decreased sexual desire or interest. Unfortunately, that is not usually what happens.

Following are some of the ways that sexual health and cancer diagnosis and treatment intersect:

- **Contraception and pregnancy:** Young adults can still become pregnant during chemotherapy and other targeted therapies, and even if somebody stops menstruating during chemotherapy, they can still get pregnant. There may be risks associated with pregnancy depending on which treatment course you are undergoing, so you will need to ask your oncology team what type of contraception is recommended given your type of cancer and treatment.

- **Treatment and sex:** Chemotherapy drugs can be found in bodily fluids, including saliva, vaginal fluids, and semen. So if you are sexually active with somebody during your chemo treatment, you can transmit those chemotherapy drugs in your bodily fluids to the other individual. I usually suggest patients wait for about seventy-two hours after each infusion before engaging in sexual activity with another person. If you still have concerns about exposing your partner, consider using a dental dam and/or condom. There also may be times during your treatment and/or chemotherapy cycle when you are at an increased risk of infection. Speak with your oncology team about specific precautions you might need to take if sexually active. Finally, there may be points in your treatment when your platelets are especially low and you are at risk of bleeding. During these times you may be asked to avoid vaginal and anal penetration due to bleeding concerns.

- **Changes in sexual function:** Some surgeries or treatments can interfere with your ability to function sexually in your preferred way. Understandably, if you've had surgery that involves part of your body traditionally associated with sexuality—such as the removal of your uterus or one or both breasts, or some colorectal procedures—it can be impactful. However, some other situations that *don't* seem immediately connected—such as if you lose a limb, or have a head and neck cancer that impacts your ability to produce saliva or move your tongue—could also interfere with sexual activity. No matter what the situation, if you have noticed any changes in sexual function that concern you, ask your team about available rehabilitation options.

- **Physical changes and body image:** In addition to hair loss, there are myriad other physical changes you can go through during cancer treatment—including weight gain, weight loss, and fluctuations in your muscle mass or tone. Chemotherapy can impact your skin and give you a temporary "chemo belly," while using a port can result in a scar on your chest and the base of your neck. Any of these alterations can cause you to struggle with your body image and how you identify as both a person and a sexual being.
- **Sexual health as part of overall health:** You can't look at your sexual life in isolation—it's part of the whole you. So if you're struggling with your body image, anxiety, or depression, or you're scared, in pain, or unable to sleep, any or all of those could influence your sexual health. They are also all interconnected. When you're anxious, for instance, you may not get enough sleep. That, in turn, can lead to fatigue, which could then result in less interest in being sexual. One thing affects another, and so on down the line.

Beyond the side effects of treatment, numerous other variables can come into play. If you're in a relationship, then that relationship—and your partner or partners—becomes part of the equation. So will your cultural or religious views of sex, the family you grew up in and *its* take on the subject, and your prior sexual experience before your diagnosis. Everything is interconnected.

Approaching Sex after Treatment

Just as cancer has changed you in many other ways, it has likely altered your sexual life. Remember in Chapter 8 where we talked about your new normal after cancer? If we look once more at the diagram from that discussion, we are reminded that while cancer has forever changed you, who you are now is determined in part by your life *before* your diagnosis:

Normal → Cancer → New Normal*
Your new normal = your old normal + your cancer experience.

Your new normal in terms of sexuality after treatment may be different, and acknowledging the changes and possible losses is part of the coping process. Trying to understand, figure out, and accept your new normal as a sexual being is part of your *healing*.

Male-Related Sexual Health Issues Post-Treatment

The two most common issues I see male patients experience are low sexual desire and erectile dysfunction. Here's more information on both.

- **Low sexual desire:** A drop in testosterone can sometimes be a factor in sexual functioning. If a male patient shares that they have experienced a change in their sexual desire or another aspect of their sexual life, I encourage them to have their testosterone levels checked. This is usually done by asking their oncology team to check the levels via blood work, or by referring the patient to a urologist specializing in sexual health to thoroughly evaluate and address (if appropriate) testosterone therapy. Even if testosterone levels are within the "normal" range, many factors can impact desire, including fatigue, changes in body image, relationship concerns, and depression.

- **Erectile dysfunction (ED):** In terms of physical challenges, this is the most common sexual side effect experienced by men after cancer treatment. As stated earlier regarding sexual health in general, physical, psychological, and relationship variables can also play a role in ED. There are numerous methods you can try to help the physical part of ED, and you may want to ask for a consultation by a urologist with sexual health expertise to discuss the best option(s) for you. The following are some interventions that can help you manage ED:

- **Medications:** This is the first approach usually recommended to patients dealing with ED. Phosphodiesterase type-5 inhibitors (known as PDE5Is), such as Viagra and Cialis, are commonly prescribed ED meds. After you take the pill there is some variability—anywhere from thirty to sixty minutes—in terms of how quickly they take effect, and you will need some stimulation to help you get an erection. Once they start working, PDE5Is can be effective for anywhere from four to thirty-six hours (although, of course, you won't maintain an erection that entire time). Talk to your physician to gauge which ED medication is best for your needs, and consider trying them on your own before using them with a partner to see how you feel and respond physically.

- **Pelvic floor physical therapy:** This is somewhat underprescribed for ED, but it can often improve erections and is worth trying in addition to PDE5Is or if medications don't meet your expectations. Pelvic floor physical therapy can also help with other possible side effects depending on your type of cancer and treatment, such as bowel and bladder management and leakage, that can interfere with your sexual life (as well as your overall well-being). This therapy requires getting a referral from a physician and is usually covered by insurance.

- **Penile injections:** These injections, which you perform yourself, are another ED treatment that may help. While the idea of injecting something into your penis can be frightening, keep in mind that it's a very quick procedure using very fine needles. You will need a referral, after which a clinician will show you how it works and help you practice.

- **Pumps:** These are not particularly effective, but if you are uncomfortable with other options, it's a much less invasive approach to treating ED.

- **Penile implants:** For young adult patients, penile implants should only be considered if other methods for treating ED are ineffective. Implants require surgery, which can be emotionally difficult to undergo after already having gone through cancer treatment. A penile implant doesn't usually affect your ability to ejaculate and orgasm. There may be some instances (depending on your specific cancer and treatment) in which you will experience dry orgasms even after penile implant—which means you will still feel the sensation of an orgasm, but there will be no fluid ejaculated.

A multitude of factors can influence ED, including anxiety, performance anxiety (excessive fear of not performing sexually), mood changes, and relationship and communication issues. Speaking with a sexual health therapist may help, especially if the treatments detailed here are not as effective as you would like.

Female-Related Sexual Health Issues Post-Treatment

Women also experience changes in their sexual health and functioning after treatment ends. This section will explain some common issues and potential interventions to discuss with your team.

Premature Menopause

Menopause naturally occurs in those with female sexual organs by around fifty-two years old, while perimenopause may start in the mid-forties when ovaries begin to produce less hormones, estrogen levels gradually taper off, and menstrual cycles (periods) become irregular and then stop completely. But for young adults with female sexual organs, like Chloe at the start of this chapter, cancer treatment and/or surgery can result in temporary or permanent premature menopause. And, because this change happens due to cancer treatment rather than gradually and naturally, it is abrupt and sudden. Abrupt menopause can affect many different parts of your body, but we're going to focus here primarily on the sexual health and emotional components of this forced transition.

Certain chemotherapies are more likely associated with permanent menopause than others. So be sure to ask your oncology team, "Am I likely to go into menopause with this treatment regimen, and, if so, is it temporary or permanent?" Oftentimes, if it *is* temporary, your menstrual cycle will start to regulate again within six months to a year after you finish active treatment. (If you have had both your ovaries removed surgically as part of your cancer treatment, that always results in permanent menopause.)

Possible Symptoms

- **Vaginal changes:** Dryness, pain, tightness, and sometimes itching can all occur, along with reduced elasticity and tightness to the vagina. There is also often decreased blood flow, a change in sensation, and an increased likelihood of vaginal or urinary tract infections.

- **Hot flashes (flushes):** These present as sudden feelings of warmth in your upper body and most often affect the face, neck, and chest. They can first lead to sweating and then a chill once they are over.

- **Changes in mood:** Women may say they feel more irritable or more easily emotional. They can cry without being sure *why* they are crying, and sometimes become overly anxious as well.

- **Fatigue:** Women say they notice a change in their energy level, similar to the experience of those going through natural menopause in their late forties or fifties.

- **Sleep difficulties:** These can be caused by hot flashes (night sweats) as well as a general inability to sleep soundly due to disturbed sleep patterns.

- **Cognitive fog:** Women going through regular menopause may report cognitive fog, which I refer to as "menopause brain." If this happens to you as a result of premature menopause, it may be layered on top of existing chemo brain changes left over from your chemotherapy. This double whammy can leave you feeling slowed down cognitively.

- **Decreased libido (sexual desire):** There is a lot more to sexual desire than just hormones, and certainly the other issues on this list are going to wind up impacting your desire as well.

Hormone Therapy

One thing I suggest to my female patients post-treatment is that they have their hormone levels checked to see if they are indeed in premature menopause. If their levels confirm this, and their cancer is not hormone sensitive—meaning that taking systemic hormone therapy will not put them at increased risk for further disease—then I usually recommend they talk with their team about the possibility of starting such therapy. This will help with many of the side effects mentioned previously, but even *with* systematic hormone therapy, you may still experience vaginal dryness and discomfort.

Vaginal Health

Attending to your vaginal health is important for your functioning, whether or not you are sexually active. For example, vaginal dryness and loss of elasticity can cause itching and vaginal discomfort/pain, making it uncomfortable to wear tight pants, ride a bike, and undergo a gynecological exam. Good vaginal health can help with these issues, and also prevent vaginal and urinary tract infections.

Dryness and loss of vaginal stretchiness during sexual intercourse, or any type of penetration—such as with sex toys—can be very painful. This often results in avoidance of sexual intimacy—who wants to engage in a behavior that causes pain?—but attention to vaginal health can be a difference maker.

Common Supports

Moisturizing

Hormone-free vaginal moisturizer can be purchased without a prescription, either at a pharmacy or online. It should be applied internally (inside your vagina) with the applicator it comes with, as well as externally by applying some with your fingers to your vulva and clitoris. Apply it every other night, before bed, so it becomes part of your bedtime routine and also so that it has time to be absorbed while you sleep and doesn't leak out. Usually after twelve weeks you will start noticing a difference.

Some moisturizers I recommend include Replens, Good Clean Love Restore, Hydro GYN, and Revaree. Sometimes you need to try a couple until you find the one you like. If over-the-counter moisturizers don't work well enough, and you're still encountering vaginal pain and dryness, consider speaking with your oncology team about getting prescribed a **local topical hormonal moisturizer**. This may not be an option, depending on your type of cancer and treatment, but it's worth asking. Prescription topical estrogen treatments come in different formulations, and your gynecologist can help you choose which is right for you. Discuss how best to apply the topical estrogen internally as well as externally to avoid itchiness and tissue shrinkage.

If you are going to be sexually intimate, you may also want to use a **lubricant**. A lot of the same companies that make over-the-counter moisturizers make lubricants as well, but be sure to read the labels carefully so you get the right product for the right use. You may want to try different lubricants to see which works best. It should be spread liberally, internally and externally, on both your vagina and anything that will be penetrating it—whether that is a penis or a sex toy. You could try applying lubricant as part of your sex play, foreplay, and love making so that it feels less intrusive and more part of the experience. Some of the lubricants I often suggest include Good Clean Love: Almost Naked Organic Lubricant, Astroglide, Sliquid, and PINK water. Again, you may want to try different options until you find the one you like best.

Pelvic Floor Physical Therapy

Pelvic floor therapy involves exercises that help you recognize when your vaginal muscles are contracting and how to relax them. They do require a referral and your insurance will cover them. It's important to work with a physical therapist who specializes in pelvic floor exercises. Usually the exercises will involve some type of internal manual therapy to help relax the muscles and aid in vaginal openness. Your physical therapist may give you a set of dilators that will help you in stretching your vagina and learning how to not tighten up as much during (or in anticipation of) penetration. This is important not only for sexual reasons but also helpful for bladder control and your ability to have comfortable gynecological examinations.

In addition, if you've had painful vaginal penetration in the past, your muscles probably have contracted (or tightened) as a reflex response to the pain. As this has continued over time, it has likely developed into a conditioned response; each time you even anticipate any type of vaginal penetration, your muscles unconsciously tense up—causing more pain and discomfort when the penetration occurs. It is similar to what happens when you're about to get a needle shot. The nurse tells you to relax, but you often subconsciously tense up anyway in anticipation of the pain—thereby tensing your arm muscles and making the shot hurt more. With vaginal penetration, the accumulation of painful experiences can lead to avoiding sexual intimacy for fear of getting hurt—which, in turn, may lead to less sexual desire.

Vibrator Therapy

Using a vibrator can be helpful for improving blood flow to your vagina. In addition, by using a vibrator yourself, you can explore what does and doesn't feel good. Ask yourself: "Has my sensation changed from before cancer?" "How has it changed?" Later, if you have a partner, you may want to share what you've discovered about what gives you pleasure.

Additional Considerations
- **Check your medications.** Allergy meds, for instance, may not only dry up the mucus in your nose but also dry up your vaginal tissue.
- **Avoid potential irritants.** These can include feminine hygiene sprays, perfumed soaps, and deodorant panty liners.

Post-Treatment Sexuality When Dating

As we know, one of the challenges of being diagnosed with early onset cancer is that this time period is when you may be just starting to explore yourself and your sexuality. In addition, you may be very nervous about dating post-treatment because of what you've gone through. Will potential partners be intimidated by the situation and bolt? Dating is already scary enough; your cancer backstory makes it that much more complicated. I like to remind young adults that *everyone* has a backstory, and nobody's life is perfect. I then explore with them whether they want to date, and if so how best to approach it; I will even help them set up profiles on dating sites.

Writing a New Script

Not surprisingly, most patients who discuss dating in our sessions want to discuss when, and *how*, they should tell people about their cancer. First, I note that every situation is different, and there is no correct answer to the *when*. In some instances cancer comes up early in the dating process, while other times it comes later. I recommend patients go slow and see how they feel with a person, and only share their situation when they feel comfortable doing so. Unless it is very obvious, there should be no pressure to open up on a first date. In terms of *how*, I encourage them to create their own scripts of what they want to say about their cancer, and then we work together on how they may wish to share it. Once they figure out exactly what they want to say, we run through it like a play rehearsal. Not just the words, but how they are communicating them—their tone, their facial expression, everything.

Patient Voices

"Breast cancer wrecked my sex life. Overnight menopause, scars, and dysmorphia hijacked my confidence and shut down my desire. Intimacy? 'It's not you, it's me—and my missing estrogen, one numb nipple, and mental spiral.' Sex used to be spontaneous, effortless, and fun. Now I'm stuck trying to manufacture desire that used to come naturally. It's messy with

lube, layered with grief, and full of reminders—like no sensation in my breasts and a body I barely recognize. It's not enough to just survive. Being alive isn't enough—I want to feel alive too."
—Christy G.

If you have similar jitters around dating, consider writing out your own script, practicing it with a close friend, and getting their honest opinions about it. This approach may seem a bit, well, scripted—but I've seen it work many times. You'll not only find the words that sound the most natural to you, but you will likely also start feeling more confident—and less afraid—about saying them.

Keep in mind that revealing your situation might not necessarily be your choice when dating. If you shared your cancer experience publicly online, there is the possibility that any of your potential matches might come across it with a simple search of your name. If they do, and you find out when starting to share your cancer news that they already know about it, well, that's pretty cool. You've found out right off the bat that they are probably *not* the type who will abandon you in tough times.

Enhancing Your Sexual Intimacy

The following are some general thoughts and suggestions about possible ways to enhance your sexual life:

- **Don't believe the movies.** Hollywood often portrays the "perfect" date as one starting with a big, romantic dinner and wine and ending with passionate sex in bed—or on a more exotic locale like the beach or kitchen table. While this might seem like an ideal option, it really isn't. I'm not sure about you, but after a big meal, most people I know feel like beached whales, ready to go to bed to digest their food. Besides, alcohol interferes with the ability of both men and women to orgasm—and can worsen vaginal dryness. The Hollywood scenario just doesn't work for most, and as someone with cancer-related issues, you may need to imagine and enjoy other scenarios better geared to your situation. If heavy meals aren't agreeing with your treatment, for instance, opt for tea and cookies in an off-the-beaten-path café. If nighttime is not the right time for you energy-wise, make the date earlier in the day. Keep in mind that during the beginning of a relationship, filled with magical and intoxicating feelings, desire seems almost automatic. But usually, as relationships grow longer lasting, desire needs nurturing to maintain.

- **Communicate and open up.** The key to intimacy and desire is open communication. If cancer has led to a change in your sex life, your partner(s) will likely be wondering about the cause. If you don't explain that this is happening because of your treatment— or because you're struggling with how you're feeling physically or due to body image issues—they won't know. Remember, while your partner(s) might also be scared and curious, they may refrain from talking or inquiring because they don't want to be insensitive. So as difficult as it is, *you* have to be the one to initiate those conversations. While it's hard to be vulnerable and talk about sex so openly, in this case it is critically important.

- **Continue cuddling.** Most people enjoy the closeness that comes with being gently touched by someone they love or care deeply for, even if they're not feeling well. So while you may feel so lousy during active treatment that you have no interest in sexual intimacy, that doesn't mean you might not both want—and enjoy—some physical closeness. Try cuddling or holding hands with your partner. Let them massage your feet.

- **Keep a desire diary.** As you are recovering, and notice that you're feeling better, try and track your energy and desire. When do you feel the most relaxed? The most likely to be interested in sexual intimacy? By keeping a diary of your feelings, as well as what feels good to you now, you can start to explore for yourself when your desire is more likely to emerge.

- **Change the focus.** Rather than setting a specific goal for intimacy, such as having an orgasm, make it about what feels good *in each moment*. If you have an orgasm, that's great, but it need not be the goal. Try making it simply about pleasure from that closeness. This can be a critically important step to rekindling desire. Be sure to explain such a change in focus to your partner(s).

- **Take your time.** When taking steps toward resuming sexual intimacy with your partner(s), it's important to give yourself time to get in the mood and relax. That may mean watching an erotic movie together or on your own, or reading some erotic literature to each other or alone—whatever works for you. You may want to listen to music, and dance, and kiss, and that's *all*. Even if it does not lead to more right now, you're still sharing a moment of intimacy.

  Progress at a pace that feels comfortable for you as an individual and as a couple. If there is going to be sexual touching, it's very important to make sure it's gentle initially, and if there are parts of your body you are not comfortable with having touched, say so. Also communicate with your partner(s) about what feels good and what doesn't. You may need extra time for foreplay, and should be ready to stop if anything feels painful or uncomfortable. Remind your partner(s) you are still adjusting to changes yourself.

- **Be careful with supplemental herbs.** A lot of people ask me about using different herbs to enhance some aspects of their sexual lives. I'd be very careful about doing this without speaking to your oncology team. Memorial Sloan Kettering Cancer Center has a free app that provides information about herbs and supplements, possible interactions, research to support their various uses, and when to avoid them. See the Resources section for more information.

- **Dare to explore.** Try self-stimulation and learn what feels good to you now. Use a vibrator. Keep an open mind when it comes to sexual pleasure. Sometimes the sexual position that gave you the most pleasure before cancer no longer works as well, and you may need to try a different position or positions. For example, women may feel more comfortable being on top during sexual intercourse now, because it provides them some control over the degree of penetration. Perhaps explore an adult sex store? Allow yourself to experiment, and try to have fun with it. Sometimes when you are too serious, you get more anxious, and that interferes with enjoyment.

Remember, your sexual health is part of your overall health and well-being. You're getting to know your body again, and processing emotionally all that you have been through. Give yourself time to acknowledge any losses, find strategies to cope with changes and/or losses, and then keep sex in perspective. You may not have the exact same sexual life as you did prior to cancer, but it can still be fulfilling and satisfying.

Key Points

- Sexual health is part of your overall health and well-being. Cancer treatment affects almost all aspects of your body and mind—and that includes your sexual life. Though sexual changes during and after cancer treatment are not always brought up by your oncology team, you need to advocate and ask them about what to expect.
- Multiple factors can impact your sexual life besides cancer treatment, such as changes in body image, anxiety, depression, fatigue, other medications you may be taking, prior sexual experiences, and your upbringing and cultural and/or religious views on sex.
- Issues like erectile dysfunction, decreased sexual desire, and premature menopause are common during and after cancer treatment, along with symptoms such as vaginal dryness,

decreased elasticity, and painful vaginal penetration. There are support options available for all of these situations.

- You'll likely experience a new normal in your sexual life, and exploring new strategies and being open and honest with yourself and your partner(s) will help you adjust and manage changes. You may want to rethink when and how to be intimate—such as earlier in the day, or with less emphasis or expectations around sex—so that cancer-related challenges like less energy or less desire don't prevent you from enjoying the closeness.

- If you are dating, it's a good idea to think ahead of time about how, when, and what you'll tell partners about your cancer. Working with a psychotherapist or a good friend and creating a script about how to approach these conversations may help.

CHAPTER 10
Living with Chronic Cancer

Glenn had been diagnosed with stage III colon cancer and successfully treated when he was forty-five. He had a busy career in finance and a great marriage and enjoyed coaching his son's soccer team. A marathoner when younger, Glenn still found time to run the occasional 5K and golf.

"Cancer was definitely tough, but I figured I was *tougher*," says Glenn. "Friends of mine who were interning in the Twin Towers died on 9/11, so I knew everything could be gone in an instant. I was getting all I could out of life."

That attitude was put to the test three years later, when Glenn learned the cancer had metastasized to one of his lungs. He was shocked and devastated, and even the assurance that treatment could control the situation provided little solace.

"My oncologist said they could remove a single nodule from my lung, start me on targeted treatment, and I could continue living with cancer," recalls Glenn. "I didn't believe him. I loved my job and the camaraderie of my colleagues, but I was ready to quit immediately and get my affairs in order."

This is when I first met Glenn. We discussed that while there was nothing wrong with preparing for worst-case scenarios, there was also no reason to stop doing what he loved. Since he had been at the same company for years, he decided to talk to his boss about more flexible hours for those days he wasn't feeling his best due to treatment. Through our conversations, Glenn realized that it was better to approach his cancer as a chronic illness rather than a terminal one.

Two years later came another setback: The cancer advanced to Glenn's liver, and he had to change his treatment. The new protocol was far more taxing, leading to fatigue, chemo brain, intractable nausea, and other side effects. Once again, we strategized around the situation; even part-time work was now difficult, so Glenn decided to go on disability. He also connected with the palliative care team, which prescribed medications and provided referrals to integrative therapies to help with the side effects. Weekly acupuncture and therapeutic massage sessions at the center were particularly beneficial, as was his daily meditation at home.

"Keeping busy was crucial, because I knew if I had too much free time, I'd just ruminate about the cancer," says Glenn. "I started cooking classes with my wife and kept on coaching my son's teams—only this time as an assistant. Giving up running and sometimes not having energy to get around the golf course was hard, but therapy gave me a space to explore my frustrations and fears about the future."

A New Kind of Panic

This chapter focuses on living with cancer that is initially diagnosed as metastatic, or that has recurred/relapsed after you have completed what seemed for a period like successful treatment.

Understanding the Terms "Relapse," "Recurrence," and "Metastasize"

Let's start by explaining some terms.

- **Metastasize:** Some people are diagnosed initially with cancer that has already metastasized, or spread, to another part of their body. Other times, people who have been treated for a cancer can have it return and spread/metastasize to another part of the body.
- **Recur(rence):** Some patients are diagnosed with localized cancer, and then at some point later on—after surgery or other treatment has "eradicated" the cancer—it returns, or recurs. It may come back in the same spot or metastasize to a different part of the body.

- **Relapse:** With blood cancers, like leukemia, we usually use the word "relapse" rather than "recurrence" to describe a cancer that has come back, but the two terms are often used interchangeably.

Some Cancers That Spread or Return Are Treated with "Curative Intent"

People often assume that when cancer recurs/relapses or metastasizes, it means they will have to live the rest of their lives being on and off treatment. It's important to clarify something right away: Not *all* cancers that recur/relapse or metastasize are "incurable."

For example, some types of metastatic testicular cancer are still treated with curative intent. So is relapsed Hodgkin lymphoma. Even if your particular cancer comes back and/or metastasizes and moves to a different part of your body, do *not* assume that it is no longer "curable." Become informed. Talk to your oncology team, and consider getting a second opinion as well. You don't necessarily *have to* do that, but it's certainly something to think about.

Here are two examples from my own experience that illustrate the value of being informed. In the early 1990s, a group of patients with advanced metastatic breast cancer were told they had no treatment options left. Then, suddenly, a clinical trial opened for a new drug called Herceptin that targeted one of the most aggressive forms of breast cancer. My patients who qualified and enrolled had such amazing responses that decades later they are *still* on Herceptin—leading engaging, productive lives with minimal side effects.

It was a similar story for some of my early young adult patients with chronic myelogenous leukemia (CML). Because CML usually occurs in older patients, for many years the life expectancy for young adults with the disease was uncertain. Then, in 1998, researchers unveiled a drug called Gleevec that was able to put patients into remission. Those who had been preparing for end of life rushed to join the first clinical trial for Gleevec, and years later—like the long-term survivors on Herceptin—some of these patients remain alive.

Why is it so vital that these points be made—and stories told—up front? It is because in my experience, people who hear that a cancer has returned or spread to elsewhere in their body tend to get extremely scared, which is understandable. In many ways, the fear and panic they felt upon their initial diagnosis comes back along with the cancer—and at times it's even worse. Their reaction is in large part due to what they see portrayed on film and television or hear from other people, which is that if the cancer comes back, forget it. At times, however, that is not the case. There are actually several different scenarios that can result from a cancer recurrence:

- Your cancer is treated again, either with the same or a different treatment plan, and you are deemed "NED" (no evidence of disease) or designated back into remission.
- Your cancer is treated again and *not* initially put into remission, and you go through several treatments before going into remission/NED.
- Your cancer is treated again and put back into remission/NED. It recurs/metastasizes at a later time, and again you try treatment(s) to go into remission or control the cancer.
- Your cancer is treated again and not initially put into remission, and you go through several treatments before going into remission/NED. It recurs/metastasizes at a later time and again you try treatment(s) to go into remission/NED or control the cancer.
- Your cancer is treated again, and the cancer is controlled but still there. If it starts to grow again or metastasizes, then treatment may be changed as your team looks for a better way to manage or hopefully have your cancer go into remission/NED.

With the last three scenarios, your oncology team will devise a plan to contain and treat your cancer as a "chronic illness," hopefully for extended periods of time—sometimes even years and decades when you are on either continuous treatment(s) or on and off treatment with some breaks. With some new treatments today, there may be patients who, after years of going on and off, find an option that might put them in a situation where they are in remission or NED for very long periods of time—and may start to feel they are "cured."

One final scenario is that your cancer is neither able to be controlled and managed nor put into remission/NED. There are no more treatment options available. In these situations, you can work with your team to focus on symptom management and quality of life and also explore options including palliative care and hospice (this is covered in more detail later in this chapter).

Cancer As a Chronic Illness

The emotional situation for individuals living with metastatic, recurrent, or relapsed (MRR) cancer is different than for those who are at early stages after diagnosis. When I encounter people with MMR, and it feels appropriate, I like to discuss with them the importance of looking at their situation more as living with a chronic illness—since the cancer is not necessarily viewed as "curable." I point out that there are many chronic illnesses that people can live with for many years, on and off treatment, such as diabetes, heart disease, and human immunodeficiency virus (HIV). So while they may still need to be on cancer treatment much of the time, I try to reassure them that they can hopefully live for a long time as well.

A big part of my therapy with these patients is focusing on *acceptance*—learning to live with being on and off treatment and shifting away from a curative to a chronic situation. Acceptance does not mean you like the situation or are fine with it, but it does mean acknowledging the reality of it. I often say, "As long as there are treatments, there is hope."

Living with Cancer

A growing number of young adults are now living with cancer and looking at it as a chronic illness. This trend toward a new type of survivorship is happening more and more. Because of treatments now available, such as targeted therapies and immunotherapies, people are living longer and better with MRR cancer.

It is a situation not unlike what has happened with HIV. People who were diagnosed with HIV in the 1980s very quickly contracted AIDS and died, but then new drugs came out, and today people are living for many years with HIV. Similarly, many types of cancer that in the past became advanced and terminal quickly—such as lung cancer and melanoma—are now much more treatable. Even if they recur or metastasize, people can have years and sometimes decades of additional survivorship.

Patient Voices

"Cancer destroyed my self-confidence, and I don't mean the confidence to wear an outfit on a Friday night, but the confidence I had in my beliefs and decision-making skills. I was confident that my work mattered and that it was what I contributed to society. When my career was interrupted by my diagnosis, I felt inconsequential. Survivorship has forced me to work on my identity and self-worth in a way I hadn't before. Who am I? No, really, who am I?" —Valerie L.

Again, a Forgotten Group

The majority of research and writing about cancer survivorship is focused on initial treatment with curative intent. There is much less emphasis on living with metastatic or relapsed disease, and what it's like to deal with years of on-again, off-again treatment; close monitoring; and frequent follow-ups at the cancer center. Even when this situation *is* addressed, there is very little on the topic as it relates to young adults—especially any mention of the constant life milestone interruptions that can occur for this group. Understandably, young adults who come to me with MRR cancer are often worried they will never be in sync with their peers or live "normal" lives due to delays in their personal, educational, and professional milestones.

Part of the frustration stems from the fact that survivorship programs are not geared to help those living with long-term or recurrent cancers, and books and journal articles on relapsed disease focus primarily on terminal disease and end-of-life care. When it comes to cancer as a chronic illness, where you hope to live for many years on and off treatment, there is very little detail on this experience—and how it impacts you emotionally, physically, and psychologically. Cancer survivors living this reality have understandably felt left out and uncertain about how to navigate their journeys. This chapter aims to fill some of that gap and provide some hopefully helpful insights.

Meeting MRR Challenges

As stated earlier, it can often be harder for young adults to deal with cancer the second time around. The immediate threat of death with MRR disease feels stronger, and your hope takes a big hit. If your first time navigating cancer was filled with complications, the thought of putting yourself and your loved ones through that roller-coaster ride again can be very distressing, even if you now have the wisdom of experience. The mainstream view of metastatic or relapsed cancer as a terminal disease—and a quick killer—does not help matters.

Following are some common issues you may have to grapple with as an MRR cancer survivor.

Long Gaps Between Diagnoses

While joining the two-time cancer club and the uncertainty that comes with membership is an adjustment for anybody, it can be particularly shocking if there has been a long gap between your cancer diagnoses. In a moment you go from thinking that you're cured and are living your life cancer-free to believing that the disease will be with you for *the rest of your life*. I've had young adult patients whose cancer has recurred ten or even twenty years after their initial diagnosis, by which point they've long since moved on personally and professionally. They've graduated from school, built careers, gotten married, had kids, and put cancer completely in their rearview mirrors. Now, in an instant, it's right back in front of them—and that can be jarring.

If you are facing cancer for a second time, and feeling this type of elevated anxiety and fear, it is helpful to talk to your oncology team. Because you may be at a different point in life than at your first diagnosis, the coping strategies you used then might not be as effective this time around. Let your team educate you about the various treatment options, and seek mental health support around how to cope with your emotions and living with cancer.

Constant Uncertainty

One thing I tell all my patients with MRR cancers is that as long as there are treatments available to them, there is hope. You need to remember that too. It may require a major psychological shift, because you need to go from thinking about being *rid* of your cancer to dealing with it all the time. Constant uncertainty, and a fear for your mortality, may also be much more present in your mind. As more time passes, you will have moments where you are able to deal with it better. I've heard from some patients who, after going from one treatment to another for a while, have times on therapy when it almost starts to feel routine—like a regular part of their lives. You will never lose that fear of dying, but over time it may go from being prominently at the forefront of your thoughts to temporarily receding to the back of your mind, depending on where you are in your treatment course.

Strain on Others

Of course, you are not the only one who will be dealing with your MRR situation. Those closely connected to you—romantic partner(s), children, family, friends, classmates, and colleagues—will also be impacted. Dealing with more treatments and potential side effects will surely be traumatic for them as well, and affect them in different ways depending on your relationships.

You may feel a sense of guilt or anxiety around having to put those in your life through "all this" again, but try to focus your precious energy on making sure they get professional help if they need it. In addition, as you develop coping strategies for the days ahead, try and help them do the same—and figure out how best to meet the challenges together. That may mean readjusting your strategies, as well as your expectations, as new issues emerge.

Unlike with your initial treatment, which had a clear end point, your approach for handling cancer as a chronic illness may have no finish line. Most cancer centers have support programs for caregivers, and sometimes even specifically for caregivers of young adult patients with MRR disease. Programs on parenting while living with chronic cancer are becoming more easily available. Ask your oncology team and social worker about them.

All Types of Cancer-Related Fatigue

Periods of physical, emotional, and cognitive fatigue can be more prevalent—and challenging—when facing MRR disease. This is due to the on-again, off-again nature of treatment. While you may get breaks between different therapy cycles or regimens during which you start to recover physically, once you get back on treatment, the fatigue will likely recur.

Spending years in this treatment pattern could result in your never *fully* getting past your fatigue, and it may become more of a chronic treatment-related weariness that you struggle to find ways to adjust to and compensate for. Some of the same strategies discussed in Chapters 4 and 8 can still be beneficial, such as moving/exercise, eating well, drinking plenty of fluids, acupuncture, therapeutic massage, and pacing yourself.

Pain

For many of my patients living with long-term chronic cancer, new pain serves as an immediate alarm—a sign that their disease has advanced. Make sure to speak with your oncology team about it. While each emergent pain and discomfort does *not* necessarily signal the presence of more cancer, it is always key to report and investigate.

One thing I routinely ask patients with pain to do is rate it on a scale of zero to ten (with ten being the worst). If their pain is at a five or above, hopefully they have already communicated it to someone on their team. The goal is to keep your pain level as low as possible, hopefully below three or four. What patients often don't realize, however, is that chronic pain can be extremely debilitating even if it is not so high on the scale. A pain level of three or four that is unrelenting and without relief can drain you of all your emotional and physical energy.

It takes a lot to deal and cope with ongoing pain, even if it is lower grade. I like to use the analogy of a low-level headache or toothache. Even after just a couple of hours, that type of nagging pain can be exhausting—and leave you unable to function at your best. Pain should be addressed and treated at any level. There is no reason in today's era of medicine that anyone should suffer; no matter what your level of pain, bring it up to your team and advocate for appropriate pain management.

Unfortunately, with all the media attention on addiction tied to pain medications, patients often fear this outcome when prescribed such meds. Cancer patients without a prior history of addiction, however, do not typically become "addicted" as long as they are taking the medications under the care of their oncology and/or pain-management/palliative care teams. Even if you have a history of substance use, you can—and still should—be treated for cancer pain. If you have concerns, talk with your oncology team.

Side Effects

While great advances have been made in emerging treatments like targeted therapies and immunotherapies, they still have side effects. Part of dealing with MRR cancer is learning to manage those side effects on an ongoing basis so you can continue to maximize your ability to engage in and enjoy life. This can be very challenging, because side effects serve as constant reminders of all you're going through, but the more you learn how to handle them, the less disruptive they may feel. Palliative care, which is discussed later in this chapter, is crucial to help with pain and symptom management.

Financial Challenges

Most young adults with MRR cancer will need to take time off from work or school. Sometimes this may be just for short periods, while in other cases it can be permanent. Usually fatigue (physical, emotional, and/or cognitive) is the biggest reason for such absences, and you may need to take numerous periodic breaks as you go on and off different treatment regimens. It can definitely be a disruption, so communicating with your employer or school administrators is important. Communicating and getting support from your medical team can help you fight for and secure disability benefits (more on that later in this section).

It's challenging to set goals and advance in your professional life—or complete the requirements needed to get an undergraduate or graduate degree—when you can't predict how you're going to feel from one week, month, or year to the next. As a result, you may find it hard to finish school, move up the ladder at work, or even keep a steady job while continuing to live with cancer. When combined with the costs associated with treatment, a sporadic work life can result in financial toxicity (distress). If you find yourself in such a situation, don't suffer in silence. Ask your clinical team about financial resources and assistance that may be available to cancer patients at your treatment center or in your community. There are also national organizations that can help, some of which are listed in the Resources section at the end of this book.

Disability Dilemmas

Many of my young adult patients struggle with the thought of taking disability leaves from their jobs, because they see it as a type of defeat—and yet another sign that they are falling behind their peers. Even if they don't feel well enough yet to return to their jobs, the thought of *not* working is scary. Cancer may be an obstacle, but not one they want to define or derail them. Besides, what if their treatment lasts for years? How are they going to save for their future or possibly help support a family, even with disability coverage? How are they going to fill their days?

The flip side of this problem is when you're *not* feeling good enough yet to return to work, and insurance/disability companies start questioning the situation—without understanding all the physical, emotional, cognitive, and psychological issues you are still dealing with due to your cancer. Patients show me letters from disability companies that read along the lines of, "We've seen you have been off treatment for six months, and your scans show your disease is stable. When will you be returning to work?"

In cases like these, I remind patients that even if their cancer is stable, or there is no evidence of disease, that does not mean that it has gone away. When you have MRR cancer, the chances are that it's coming back again eventually. Besides, while you may not be on active treatment *now*, you could be coming off three years straight where you *were*. You should only go back to work if and when you feel up to it.

If a situation arises where you are being threatened with removal of your disability coverage, I've learned through experience what might be the culprit. When social security, disability, and/or insurance companies receive the notes from your oncologist, they focus on the most recent information. If your neuroendocrine tumor is currently under control, for instance, the note might state, "Patient doing better. No evidence of disease." This is not indicative, of course, of all that's *really* going on. So I often suggest to patients that they ask their oncology teams to write summary notes to social security and/or the disability companies explaining the *overall* oncology situation and that they are living with cancer (even if it is temporarily not visible on scans).

Also, if you are working with a mental health professional such as a social worker, psychiatrist, or psychologist, ask if they will advocate on your behalf by writing a letter to the disability company detailing your challenges living with chronic cancer—including fatigue, cognitive issues, and (if applicable) premature menopause. Have them cite research if possible.

At times, you may be referred by social security and/or the disability company to their own mental health professional. These clinicians usually have no background whatsoever in oncology—which, naturally, can impact their analysis. For example, if they valuate a cancer patient for signs of depression, they won't understand that high levels of anxiety are often expected with MRR disease. They also don't know about cancer-related fatigue and/or cognitive impairment. In cases like this, I will often intervene and contact the mental health provider myself or write a letter to explain and educate them on psychosocial oncology.

Remember, as a person living with chronic cancer, you are dealing with the effects of being on prolonged treatment with numerous side effects that will impact you across all realms of your life. The effects of these challenges do not simply go away when you go off treatment, whether that's for one month, three months, six months, or even a year or more. Recovery takes significant time, and it is important that you get the help you are entitled to and need. Asking your treatment team to support your requests or claims to companies can help make this happen.

The Liability of Looking Good

As you continue living with MRR cancer, you may find yourself going through stretches between treatments when you look very good externally. Your hair grows back, your color returns, and you regain your appetite—along with some weight. Which is all good, right?

Well, not quite. The challenge comes when you start hearing the same refrain from seemingly everybody you meet: "Wow, you look terrific! It's hard to believe you have cancer!" However well intentioned, such comments can also be troubling. Hear them often enough, and you may start wondering why you're *not* feeling as terrific as you look. While the reason could be very legitimate—perhaps you're in the midst of a new immunotherapy protocol—you may be too embarrassed to disclose the truth: You're so tired you can barely keep your head up, but you've learned to pace yourself and go out just for short periods.

What these well-wishers can't know from a quick glance is that beneath your shirt you might have skin rashes you've been grappling with for months. You may be forever looking for the nearest restroom because of the diarrhea that comes without warning, or worrying about thyroiditis, hepatitis, pneumonitis, and any other "itises" you can think of. Then there is the mental exercise of accepting that you have a chronic and incurable disease, one capable of throwing any number of curveballs your way at any time.

It can all be frustrating, but you *do* have some control over your own cancer narrative. You can choose to educate others on the reality you are living, or choose not to do so. It's your decision how much you want to share about what lies beneath.

Isolation and Spiritual Distress

When you were initially diagnosed, you might have thought along the lines of, "Okay, I may be somewhat isolated during treatment, and for a while as I recover, but eventually I'll find a way to reintegrate with my peers. It may take a year, or even *two*, but that's the hope." Now, with the constant interruptions and disruptions that come from being repeatedly on and off active treatment, you can feel more alone than ever— with even fewer people who understand what you are going through.

Living with cancer as a chronic illness takes a toll. It may, unfortunately, fall on you to educate others about your lived reality. Participating in programs for those with chronic cancer and their families can be extremely valuable. It is also vitally important, if you have or live with young children of an appropriate developmental stage, that you inform *them* about your situation. They should understand the reason you may be fatigued or not feeling well is due to treatment for the cancer. The same communication strategies discussed in earlier chapters apply here. At Dana-Farber and other cancer centers, there are programs and groups specifically for people living with ongoing cancer, including using meaning-centered therapy (developed at Memorial Sloan Kettering Cancer Center by William S. Breitbart, MD), a psychotherapeutic intervention focused on helping patients find purpose and well-being in the midst of a serious medical challenge.

Similarly, while it may have been helpful to lean on your spirituality after your initial diagnosis, you may now be in a sort of spiritual distress, wondering, "How can this be happening to me *again*?" There is no easy answer, but how you face this new situation can help you cope. If you are inclined, this may be an ideal time to speak with either the chaplain at your cancer center and/or the leader(s) at your own institution of worship.

Finding Balance Living with Chronic Cancer

A lot of my work with patients facing MRR cancer involves helping them try to find a balance between staying hopeful and living with the reality of recurrent cancer. Finding that balance is tough, and what I find is that most people tend to fluctuate, which is a normal and expected response to a changing health situation. For example, some might think: "I'm really trying to be hopeful that this treatment will work, but if it doesn't, I'll just have to readjust to a new one."

This patient does not know if their current treatment is going to stabilize the cancer. They certainly want to *believe* it will, but they are worried—perhaps it's a new therapy without a long track record yet. So they are trying to stay cautiously optimistic, and while they don't know the virtues of the next option down the line either, they plan to be ready for it if necessary.

When talking with young adults as they are working toward adjusting to cancer as a chronic illness, I also hear things like: "When I was initially diagnosed, I was told that this should be it—they'd be able to get rid of the tumor for good. It was unusual to develop cancer at such a young age, but I accepted it and went in expecting to be cured. I had hope, I *focused* on that hope, and they said the cancer was gone. Now it's come back. The unexpected has happened not once, but *twice*, and I'm having to deal with cancer all over again. How can I get back to that place of hope, given that these crazy things keep happening to me? I'm scared, and don't want to get too hopeful only to then get disappointed."

Again, it's really about trying to find that balance while realizing you can feel two or more emotions simultaneously. That's a lot of what we do in therapy. Sometimes, when a treatment works for a long period, patients are able to stay cautiously optimistic for longer periods of time. Your hope and concerns travel side by side.

Accepting the Unknown

A lot of the young adults I see with MRR cancers tell me they struggle with making long-term plans because they never know what's going to happen. They may *think* that they are doing well, but then the day of their three-month scan approaches, and they start getting extremely anxious. Their hope is to live from one scan to another without being consumed by fear, and we work together on being flexible with their planning. That may mean more short-term rather than long-term plans, or taking precautions like buying vacation insurance for a trip away in case they need to cancel at the last moment. The same strategies we discussed regarding coping with FCR (fear of cancer recurrence) in Chapter 8 work in this situation as well.

Living with chronic cancer is unpredictable and usually has no finish line. You don't know *if* it's going to go away, and when (or if) it might come back. Because of this unpredictability, MRR cancer has the potential to derail your goals. Your challenge is to try and keep your train on its tracks by taking care of your overall well-being and using the strategies we have discussed to focus on what gives your life purpose—even if it's only for moments each day.

In some ways it's really about accepting the unknown. Cancer may continue disrupting your life, and your resulting anger or frustration is justified. You may continue struggling to keep in sync with your peers personally and professionally. Hopefully, you try to adjust to the unwelcome changes cancer has brought and still find ways to stay engaged in living, by spending time with those you love, setting shorter-term goals, or taking fewer school classes. I have patients who took longer than they expected but still completed their degrees, took magnificent trips to exciting locales, and formed intimate and loving friendships and relationships. That doesn't mean they are happy all the time or never have moments of disappointment. It's about finding balance. Showing compassion and kindness toward yourself can go a long way in your ability to cope. Again, there is no right or wrong way.

Tips for Finding Balance

Here are some suggestions to help you find balance between acknowledging your fears and challenges while still finding joy in life.

Keep Your Key People Informed

As you continue to live with MRR cancer, you likely won't have the same level of support you did when going through your initial diagnosis and treatment. The outpouring of help and encouragement you received then was genuine, but as time goes on, people get so busy with their own lives and challenges that they lose track of the fact you are still living with cancer—especially if yours is an on-again, off-again journey. Some people may assume that you're doing fine if they don't hear from you, while others may not inquire for fear of upsetting you. Better, they think, to not broach the subject.

This should not be seen as a sign that others don't care. As we've already discussed, most people don't have a real understanding of all the physical, emotional, and logistical challenges associated with MRR cancer. By keeping a few of your key friends and family members informed about your status, either through calls or group emails/messages, you can ensure that those you are the closest to stay in the loop. Let them know that even if you *look* healthy, you're still dealing with your cancer in various ways—and open to talking about it and still needing help and support.

Get Professional Support

We've talked a lot throughout this book about using coping strategies at different points of your cancer trajectory. As you continue living with MRR disease, consider talking on a regular or semiregular basis with a mental health professional. Many of my young adult patients find it's very helpful, even when their disease is stable, to discuss the fears and uncertainties of their situations. Some do it more regularly, whether or not they are in active treatment, while others only check in during major changes in their conditions to help readjust their thinking for the challenges ahead. Do whatever feels right for you, and remember you don't need a crisis to find the best people to help you through it.

Join a Support Group for Young Adults Living with Chronic Cancer

Connecting with other young adults with MRR cancer can also be critically important, in good times and bad, because these peers are the only people who really understand all that you're going through. If you can't find the right support group near your home, consider joining one online. Your oncology team may be helpful in finding the right fit, or check out the Resources section.

Ask for Palliative Care

As discussed in Chapter 3, palliative care teams focus on keeping your quality of life as good as possible by managing your symptoms and side effects—including pain. Knowing from experience that it is easier to prevent lower-level pain from getting worse than waiting until pain becomes excruciating to deal with it, palliative care specialists can educate you on how pain management works and provide available treatment choices. They can also talk with you about your existential concerns and fears and help you review choices on practical matters like living wills and healthcare proxies.

Remember, you don't have to wait until you have pain to derive palliative care benefits. These clinicians can be a valuable part of your team right from the point of diagnosis. Anytime you have bothersome symptoms that are becoming intrusive and impacting your functioning, palliative care specialists can step in and work with your oncology group as one integrated unit.

End-of-Life Care

I will preface this section by saying that given the state of oncology care today, and the myriad treatment options and clinical trials available, it is sometimes hard to know when someone is actually entering the end-of-life phase (six months or less to live). It can become difficult in many cases to ascertain when you really *are* reaching the end of your options.

Unfortunately, there may come a time when there truly are no more alternatives. There are some outstanding books devoted entirely to end-of-life cancer care, a few of which are listed in the Resources section. They describe the struggles oncology teams often have when talking with young adults about poor prognosis and limited/lack of treatment choices, because the situation is so unjust. As hard as these discussions are for both sides, however, you deserve to hear the truth, even when it is difficult.

Some of the commonly expressed concerns by patients at end of life include fear of suffering and pain, impact on family, practical planning, quantity versus quality of life, how they want their end of life to look, and legacy. Here's a closer look at each.

Addressing Pain and Suffering

At this time, pain and suffering encompasses both physical and emotional (or existential) challenges. While physical pain can be addressed by a good palliative care/pain-management team, existential pain is much harder to handle because it can't just be treated.

For those of you with a strong spiritual and/or religious orientation, talking to your chaplain and/or religious guides can be soothing and calming. For those without that focus, seeking the counsel of mental health professionals and support groups can help you find your most comfortable path. The organization Five Wishes and the brochure "Voicing My Choices," both in the Resources section at the back of this book, can be instrumental tools in guiding these topics.

Deciding How You Want to Live

I often speak with patients about how they envision spending whatever time they have left, and if you're facing this situation you might choose to ponder the same questions I ask them: What can you still do? What is really meaningful to you? Perhaps it is watching movies with loved ones, sitting out in the sun, holding hands and sleeping with someone dear to you, eating your favorite foods, or watching your favorite sports team.

Capturing Messages for Loved Ones

In many instances, I have helped my young adult patients who are parents make videos for their own children—or others important to them. The videos are different, depending on the adults and children involved: Some are brief, sharing pearls of wisdom or guiding principles for life; others include family histories as well as thoughts on life challenges and possible ways to approach them; and still others contain more personal details such as shared memories, who the parents were as people, and their hopes and dreams for the children's future. We usually create the videos over several sessions, often in an interview format.

If you want to make one yourself but don't have a mental health provider to help in the endeavor, there is an organization called Memories Live that can work with you on creating videos for children as well as other family members. Some patients worry that such a project is a sign they are "giving up." In these instances, I tell them about several of my patients who made videos years ago, then got on clinical trials and today are still alive—and some choose to share the videos with their now adult children.

Another thing I've done is help young adult patients write cards to be given to their children or other family members on specific occasions after they are gone. This is much less labor intensive than creating a video and can still be very meaningful. Then there are many young adults who prefer not to do anything like these two options, either from lack of desire, energy, and/or time. That's fine too, of course.

Other End-of-Life Considerations

I also explore with my patients another question: What do they still have agency over? For many of them, it is making sure they have completed practical tasks such as their wills, their wishes regarding the care of their children (if they have them), and even their own funeral arrangements.

Laying the groundwork for an end-of-life event can provide you with a sense of control, as you choose details including whether you want to be buried or cremated, where to have the service or funeral, if music should be played (and if so, what), who should speak (and who should *not*), where you want to be buried, and whether you desire a religious service. Not everyone, however, gets to a point of acceptance and taking part in such activities.

There is no right or wrong way to approach end of life. You should do whatever feels right for you. After all, it is *your* life.

Assessing Quantity versus Quality of Life

Striking this balance is another thing that patients can struggle with. Some choose to stay on treatments until the very end, trying everything they can. Others, once it seems they have six months or less to live, prefer that their oncology team refer them to hospice.

With an emphasis on comfort care provided by a team, hospice care can take place either at the patient's home or in a hospice unit set up to provide comprehensive and compassionate care for patients and their families. Some people may choose to be alert while in hospice, even if that means some discomfort. Others may want to make sure their pain is totally controlled, and sleep as much as possible. I have patients who take psychedelics toward end of life, and others who have no interest. It is really up to each person to decide what feels right for them.

Leaving a Legacy

Last, I want to touch on what people leave behind after they are gone. Some people choose something very specific, such as a donation to a favorite charity or videos like those I mentioned previously. Most, however, are not as intentional. I believe that *everyone* leaves a legacy, because we all touch so many other individuals—even just in our everyday interactions through the years. Of course, you know your loved ones will remember you, but there are countless random people who you have left an impression and imprint on as well.

For nearly thirty-five years, I have had the honor to be there with many patients during this time. It is never easy. I often stay in touch with families for years after their loved ones die, and get calls when they want to share momentous life events or just talk about the person who is gone. In fact, some of the children of young adults I treated at end of life now have children of their own. Often those kids are named after their late grandparent, or have characteristics of the young adult who died. I love seeing that. It is another way that their legacy continues.

Key Points

- Sometimes cancer that has been put into remission can metastasize, relapse, or recur (MRR cancer). MRR cancer can often be treated and/or managed, and some people can go in and out of remission numerous times over a period of years or even decades.
- Thanks to new treatments and therapy options, people are living longer and better with MRR cancer as a chronic illness.
- Though parts of an MRR cancer experience are similar to an initial diagnosis and treatment, there are new and sometimes more challenging physical and emotional issues to face, from constant uncertainty to difficulty securing disability insurance. Support is available through your care team and national organizations.
- Sometimes, when all other options have been tried, end-of-life care is necessary. Even during this most difficult time, you can live with purpose and will leave a legacy.

Conclusion:
Living with Purpose

Before ending, I want to briefly share some ideas for how you can use your cancer experience as a way to enjoy a greater sense of purpose in your life.

We discussed volunteering in Chapter 6. After undergoing this huge challenge in your life—and knowing how important resources were and continue to be to your well-being—you may specifically be drawn to advocacy, a form of volunteering focused on influencing public opinion or policy changes.

Advocacy can also be a form of self-care, as it often starts with your own *personal* advocacy during the diagnostic process: asking questions, making sure you get all the tests you need, and researching treatment and recovery options. Later, you may decide to use what you've learned to advocate for others, perhaps through helping a local cancer foundation or engaging in peer-to-peer volunteering with new patients. You might even explore national cancer advocacy, which can entail meeting with leaders in Congress and elsewhere to educate them about research/clinical needs, the importance of passing cancer bills and legislation, and the allocation of funding to help others with cancer. As with all volunteering related to cancer, however, I recommend you wait a year after your treatment ends to dive in—and, when you do, don't overdo it. Pace yourself.

Of course, volunteering and advocacy are not for everyone. Each of you will find your own course to living meaningfully. Everyone is different in what brings them joy and purpose to their life. I hope this book has provided some guidance to help in this pursuit.

Patient Voices

"I started doing cancer advocacy as a way to take this terrible thing that happened to me (getting diagnosed with stage IV cancer) and make it have meaning. I continue to share my story because I've learned it makes a difference and helps make change happen. I share my story for those who may not be ready to share their own stories and for those who are no longer here to share theirs." —Bethany R.

Bibliography

Chapter 1

Adolescent and Young Adult Oncology Progress Review Group. "Closing the Gap: Research and Care Imperatives for Adolescents and Young Adults with Cancer." National Cancer Institute, August 2006. https://cancer.gov/types/aya/research/ayao-august-2006.pdf.

American Cancer Society. "ACS Cancer Treatment and Survivorship Facts & Figures 2012." American Cancer Society, 2012.

American Cancer Society. "American Cancer Society Prevention and Early Detection Guidelines." https://cancer.org/health-care-professionals/american-cancer-society-prevention-early-detection-guidelines.html.

GBD 2019 Adolescent and Young Adult Cancer Collaborators. "The Global Burden of Adolescent and Young Adult Cancer in 2019: A Systematic Analysis for the Global Burden of Disease Study 2019." *The Lancet Oncology* 23, no. 1 (2022): 27–52.

Janssen, S.H.M., W.T.A. van der Graaf, D.J. van der Meer, E. Manten-Horst, and O. Husson. "Adolescent and Young Adult (AYA) Cancer Survivorship Practices: An Overview." *Cancers (Basel)* 13, no. 19 (September 28, 2021): 4,847.

Johnson, S.B., R.W. Blum, and J.N. Giedd. "Adolescent Maturity and the Brain: The Promise and Pitfalls of Neuroscience Research in Adolescent Health Policy." *Journal of Adolescent Health* 45, no. 3 (2009): 216–21. https://doi.org/10.1016/j.jadohealth.2009.05.016.

Lewis, D.R., N.L. Seibel, A.W. Smith, and M.R. Stedman. "Adolescent and Young Adult Cancer Survival." *Journal of the National Cancer Institute Monographs* 2014, no. 49 (November 2014): 228–35.

Shek, D.T.L. "COVID-19 Pandemic and Developmental Outcomes in Adolescents and Young Adults: In Search of the Missing Links." *Journal of Adolescent Health* 69, no. 5 (2021): 683–84. https://doi.org/10.1016/j.jadohealth.2021.07.035.

Siegel, R.L., A.N. Giaquinto, and A. Jemal. "Cancer Statistics, 2024." *CA: A Cancer Journal for Clinicians* 74, no. 1 (2024): 12–49.

Tricoli, J.V., et al. "Biologic and Clinical Characteristics of Adolescent and Young Adult Cancers: Acute Lymphoblastic Leukemia, Colorectal Cancer, Breast Cancer, Melanoma, and Sarcoma." *Cancer* 122, no. 7 (2016): 1,017–28.

van der Meer, D.J., et al. "Incidence, Survival, and Mortality Trends of Cancers Diagnosed in Adolescents and Young Adults (15–39 Years): A Population-Based Study in the Netherlands 1990–2016." *Cancers (Basel)* 12, no. 11 (2020): 3,421.

Vos, T., S.S. Lim, C. Abbafati, et al. "Global Burden of 369 Diseases and Injuries in 204 Countries and Territories, 1990–2019: A Systematic Analysis for the Global Burden of Disease Study 2019." *The Lancet* 396, no. 10258 (2020): 1,204–22.

Chapter 2

Kirchhoff, A.C., A.R. Waters, A. Chevrier, and J.A. Wolfson. "Access to Care for Adolescents and Young Adults with Cancer in the United States: State of the Literature." *Journal of Clinical Oncology* 42, no. 6 (February 20, 2024): 642–52.

McDaniels-Davidson, C., et al. "Improved Survival in Cervical Cancer Patients Receiving Care at National Cancer Institute–Designated Cancer Centers." *Cancer* 128, no. 19 (October 1, 2022): 3,479–86.

Muffly, L., T.H.M. Keegan, H.Z. Mui, E.M. Alvarez, R. Siden, L.M. Holdsworth, and H.M. Parsons. "Specialized Cancer Care for Adolescent and Young Adult Acute Lymphoblastic Leukemia: Barriers and Opportunities." *Journal of the National Comprehensive Cancer Network* 23, no. 4 (2025): e247097.

Chapter 3

Burns, K., and A.W. Loren. "Fertility Preservation in Adolescents and Young Adults with Cancer: A Case-Based Review." *Journal of Clinical Oncology* 42, no. 6 (February 20, 2024): 725–34.

Clowse, M.E.B., M.A. Behera, C.K. Anders, S. Copland, C.J. Coffman, P.C. Leppert, and L.A. Bastian. "Ovarian Preservation by GnRH Agonists During Chemotherapy: A Meta-Analysis." *Journal of Women's Health* 18, no.,3 (March 2009): 311–19.

Imai, A., S. Ichigo, K. Matsunami, H. Takagi, and I. Kawabata. "Ovarian Function Following Targeted Anti-angiogenic Therapy with Bevacizumab." *Molecular and Clinical Oncology* 6, no. 6 (June 2017): 807–10.

Łubik-Lejawka, D., I. Gabriel, A. Marzec, and A. Olejek. "Oncofertility As an Essential Part of Comprehensive Cancer Treatment in Patients of Reproductive Age, Adolescents, and Children." *Cancers (Basel)* 16, no. 10 (May 13, 2024): 1,858.

McCollam, S., C. Shipman, J. Bubalo, and S. Krieg. "Preventing Chemotherapy-Induced Infertility in Female Patients." *Journal of Hematology Oncology Pharmacy* 9, no. 4 (2019): 192–98.

Smith, K.L., C. Gracia, A. Sokalska, and H. Moore. "Advances in Fertility Preservation for Young Women with

Cancer." *ASCO Educational Book*, no. 38 (May 23, 2018): 27–37.

Chapter 4

Ahles, T.A., J.C. Root, and E.L. Ryan. "Cancer- and Cancer Treatment–Associated Cognitive Change: An Update on the State of the Science." *Journal of Clinical Oncology* 30, no. 30 (2012): 3,675 –86.

Bower, J.E. "Cancer-Related Fatigue—Mechanisms, Risk Factors, and Treatments." *Nature Reviews Clinical Oncology* 11, no. 10 (October 2014): 597–609.

Jim, H.S.L., S.L. Jennewein, G.P. Quinn, D.R. Reed, and B.J. Small. "Cognition in Adolescent and Young Adults Diagnosed with Cancer: An Understudied Problem." *Journal of Clinical Oncology* 36, no. 27 (2018): 2,752–54.

Janelsins, M.C., S.R. Kesler, T.A. Ahles, and G.R. Morrow. "Prevalence, Mechanisms, and Management of Cancer-Related Cognitive Impairment." *International Review of Psychiatry* 26, no. 1 (2014): 102–13.

Morrow, G.R., P.L.R. Andrews, J.T. Hickok, J.A. Roscoe, and S. Matteson. "Fatigue Associated with Cancer and Its Treatment." *Supportive Care in Cancer* 10, no. 5 (July 2002): 389–98.

Nowe, E., Y. Stöbel-Richter, A. Sender, K. Leuteritz, M. Friedrich, and K. Geue. "Cancer-Related Fatigue in Adolescents and Young Adults: A Systematic Review of the Literature." *Critical Reviews in Oncology/Hematology* 118 (2017): 63–69.

Turgeman, I., and H. West. "Adolescents and Young Adults with Cancer." *JAMA Oncology* 9, no. 3 (2023): 440.

Chapter 5

Fox, R.S., et al. "Social Isolation and Social Connectedness among Young Adult Cancer Survivors: A Systematic Review." *Cancer* 129, no. 19 (2023): 2,946–65.

Chapter 6

Baikie, K.A., and K. Wilhelm. "Emotional and Physical Health Benefits of Expressive Writing." *Advances in Psychiatric Treatment* 11, no. 5 (2005): 338–46.

Beetz, A., K. Uvnäs-Moberg, H. Julius, and K. Kotrschal. "Psychosocial and Psychophysiological Effects of Human-Animal Interactions: The Possible Role of Oxytocin." *Frontiers in Psychology* 3 (July 9, 2012): 234.

Biggs, A., P. Brough, and S. Drummond. "Lazarus and Folkman's Psychological Stress and Coping Theory." In *The Handbook of Stress and Health: A Guide to Research and Practice*, edited by Cary L. Cooper and James C. Quick, 351–64. Chichester, UK: Wiley Blackwell, 2017.

Brickman, P., and D.T. Campbell. "Hedonic Relativism and Planning the Good Society." In *Adaptation Level Theory: A Symposium*, edited by M.H. Apley, 287–302. New York: Academic Press, 1971.

Carr, A.M., and P. Pendry. "Assessing Attendance Frequency and Duration at a Drop-In Animal Visitation Program among First-Semester University Students Separated from Their Pets." *Anthrozoös* 37, no. 1 (2023): 55–74.

Mehta, R., K. Sharma, L. Potters, A.G. Wernicke, and B. Parashar. "Evidence for the Role of Mindfulness in Cancer: Benefits and Techniques." *Cureus* 11, no. 5 (May 9, 2019): e4629.

Niles, A.N., K.E.B. Haltom, C.M. Mulvenna, M.D. Lieberman, and A.L. Stanton. "Randomized Controlled Trial of Expressive Writing for Psychological and Physical Health: The Moderating Role of Emotional Expressivity." *Anxiety, Stress, & Coping* 27, no. 1 (2014): 1–17.

Pendry, P., and J.L. Vandagriff. "Animal Visitation Program (AVP) Reduces Cortisol Levels of University Students: A Randomized Controlled Trial." *AERA Open* 5, no. 2 (2019).

Pennebaker, J.W. "Expressive Writing in Psychological Science." *Perspectives on Psychological Science* 13, no. 2 (2017): 226–29.

Ruini, C., and C.C. Mortara. "Writing Technique Across Psychotherapies—from Traditional Expressive

Writing to New Positive Psychology Interventions: A Narrative Review." *Journal of Contemporary Psychotherapy* 52, no. 1 (2022): 23–34.

Schoenmakers, E.C., T.G. van Tilburg, and T. Fokkema. "Problem-Focused and Emotion-Focused Coping Options and Loneliness: How Are They Related?" *European Journal of Ageing* 12, no. 2 (February 11, 2015): 153–161.

Stanisławski, K. "The Coping Circumplex Model: An Integrative Model of the Structure of Coping with Stress." *Frontiers in Psychology* 10 (April 16, 2019): 694.

Stefanski, V. "Social Stress in Laboratory Rats: Behavior, Immune Function, and Tumor Metastasis." *Physiology & Behavior* 73, no. 3 (June 2001): 385–91.

Zhou, E.S., and C.J. Recklitis. "Internet-Delivered Insomnia Intervention Improves Sleep and Quality of Life for Adolescent and Young Adult Cancer Survivors." *Pediatric Blood & Cancer* 67, no. 9 (June 22, 2020): e28506.

Chapter 7

American Psychiatric Association. *Diagnostic and Statistical Manual of Mental Disorders*. 5th ed. Arlington, VA: American Psychiatric Publishing, 2013.

Brothers, B.M et al. "Cognitive Behavioral Interventions." In

Psycho-Oncology, 2nd ed., 415–21. New York: Oxford University Press, 2010.

Lederberg, M.S., et al. "Supportive Psychotherapy and Cancer." In Psycho-Oncology, 3rd ed., 443–48. New York: Oxford University Press, 2015.

Lichtenthal, W.G., et al. "Meaning-Centered Psychotherapy." In Psycho-Oncology, 3rd ed., 475–79. New York: Oxford University Press, 2015.

McGrady, M.E., V.W. Willard, A.M. Williams, and T.M. Brinkman. "Psychological Outcomes in Adolescent and Young Adult Cancer Survivors." Journal of Clinical Oncology 42, no. 6 (February 20, 2024): 707–16.

Nichol, B., R. Wilson, A. Rodrigues, and C. Haighton. "Exploring the Effects of Volunteering on the Social, Mental, and Physical Health and Well-Being of Volunteers: An Umbrella Review." Voluntas (May 4, 2023): 1–32.

Osmani, V., L. Hörner, S.J. Klug, and L.F. Tanaka. "Prevalence and Risk of Psychological Distress, Anxiety, and Depression in Adolescent and Young Adult (AYA) Cancer Survivors: A Systematic Review and Meta-Analysis." Cancer Medicine 12, no. 17 (September 2023): 18,354–67.

Park, E.M., and D.L. Rosenstein. "Depression in Adolescents and Young Adults with Cancer." Dialogues in Clinical Neuroscience 17, no. 2 (June 2015): 171–80.

Pozo-Kaderman, C., and W.F. Pirl. "Depression and Anxiety Disorders in Patients with Cancer." Psychiatric Times 34, no. 3 (March 31, 2017).

Strada, E.A., and B.M. Sourkes. "Principles of Psychotherapy." In Psycho-Oncology, 2nd ed., 397–401. New York: Oxford University Press, 2010.

Traeger, L., J.A. Greer, C. Fernandez-Robles, et al. "Evidence-Based Treatment of Anxiety in Patients with Cancer." Journal of Clinical Oncology 30, no. 10 (2012): 1,197–1,205.

Chapter 8

Adams, S.C., et al. "Young Adult Cancer Survivorship: Recommendations for Patient Follow-Up, Exercise Therapy, and Research." JNCI Cancer Spectrum 5, no. 1 (October 28, 2020): pkaa099.

Barnett, M., et al. "Psychosocial Outcomes and Interventions among Cancer Survivors Diagnosed During Adolescence and Young Adulthood (AYA): A Systematic Review." Journal of Cancer Survivorship 10, no. 5 (October 2016): 814–31.

Bergerot, C.D., E.J. Philip, P.G. Bergerot, N. Siddiq, S. Tinianov, and M. Lustberg. "Fear of Cancer Recurrence or Progression: What Is It and What Can We Do about It?" American Society of Clinical Oncology Educational Book 42 (April 2022): 1–10.

Butow, P., L. Sharpe, B. Thewes, J. Turner, J. Gilchrist, and J. Beith. "Fear of Cancer Recurrence: A Practical Guide for Clinicians." *Oncology (Williston Park)* 32, no. 1 (January 15, 2018): 32–38. https://pubmed.ncbi.nlm.nih.gov/29447419/.

Crist, J.V., and E.A. Grunfeld. "Factors Reported to Influence Fear of Recurrence in Cancer Patients: A Systematic Review." *Psycho-Oncology* 22, no. 5 (May 2013): 978–86.

Fox, R.S., et al. "Social Isolation and Social Connectedness among Young Adult Cancer Survivors: A Systematic Review." *Cancer* 129, no. 19 (October 1, 2023): 2,946–65.

Hydeman, J.A., O.C. Uwazurike, E.I. Adeyemi, and L.K. Beaupin. "Survivorship Needs of Adolescent and Young Adult Cancer Survivors: A Concept Mapping Analysis." *Journal of Cancer Survivorship* 13, no. 1 (February 2019): 34–42.

Janssen, S.H.M., W.T.A. van der Graaf, D.J. van der Meer, E. Manten-Horst, and O. Husson. "Adolescent and Young Adult (AYA) Cancer Survivorship Practices: An Overview." *Cancers (Basel)* 13, no. 19 (September 28, 2021): 4,847.

Matsunaga, M., Y. He, M.T. Khine, X. Shi, R. Okegawa, Y. Li, H. Yatsuya, and A. Ota. "Prevalence, Severity, and Risk Factors of Cancer-Related Fatigue among Working Cancer Survivors: A Systematic Review and Meta-Analysis." *Journal of Cancer Survivorship* (February 28, 2024).

McGrady, M.E., V.W. Willard, A.M. Williams, and T.M. Brinkman. "Psychological Outcomes in Adolescent and Young Adult Cancer Survivors." *Journal of Clinical Oncology* 42, no. 6 (February 20, 2024): 707–16.

Neves, M.C., A. Bártolo, J.B. Prins, C.M.D. Sales, and S. Monteiro. "Taking Care of an Adolescent and Young Adult Cancer Survivor: A Systematic Review of the Impact of Cancer on Family Caregivers." *International Journal of Environmental Research and Public Health* 20, no. 8 (April 12, 2023): 5,488.

Nowe, E., et al. "Cancer-Related Fatigue in Adolescents and Young Adults: A Systematic Review of the Literature." *Critical Reviews in Oncology/Hematology* 118 (2017): 63–69.

Oldacres, L., J. Hegarty, P. O'Regan, N.M. Murphy-Coakley, and M.M. Saab. "Interventions Promoting Cognitive Function in Patients Experiencing Cancer-Related Cognitive Impairment: A Systematic Review." *Psycho-Oncology* 32, no. 2 (February 2023): 214–28.

Podina, I.R., D. Todea, and L.A. Fodor. "Fear of Cancer Recurrence and Mental Health: A Comprehensive Meta-Analysis." *Psycho-Oncology* 32, no. 10 (October 2023): 1,503–13.

Tibubos, A.N., et al. "Fatigue in Survivors of Malignant Melanoma and Its Determinants: A Register-Based Cohort Study." *Support Care Cancer* 27, no. 8 (2019): 2,809–18.

Thong, M.S.Y., et al. "Cancer-Related Fatigue: Causes and Current Treatment Options." *Oncology* 23, no. 3 (March 2022): 450–51.

Vandraas, K.F., K.V. Reinertsen, C.E. Kiserud, and H.C. Lie. "Fear of Cancer Recurrence among Young Adult Cancer Survivors—Exploring Long-Term Contributing Factors in a Large, Population-Based Cohort." *Journal of Cancer Survivorship* 15, no. 4 (August 2021): 497–508.

Yuan, X., X. Zhang, J. He, and W. Xing. "Interventions for Financial Toxicity among Cancer Survivors: A Scoping Review." *Critical Reviews in Oncology/Hematology* 192 (December 2023): 104,140.

Chapter 9

Bober, S.L., and V.S. Varela. "Sexuality in Adult Cancer Survivors: Challenges and Intervention." *Journal of Clinical Oncology* 30, no. 30 (October 20, 2012): 3,712–19.

Cherven, B.O., J. Demedis, and N.N. Frederick. "Sexual Health in Adolescents and Young Adults with Cancer." *Journal of Clinical Oncology* 42, no. 6 (February 20, 2024): 717–24.

Falk, S.J., and S. Bober. "Cancer and Female Sexual Function." *Obstetrics and Gynecology Clinics of North America* 51, no. 2 (June 2024): 365–80.

Falk, S.J., and S. Bober. "Vaginal Health During Breast Cancer Treatment." *Current Oncology Reports* 18, no. 5 (May 2016): 32.

Frederick, N.N., C.J. Recklitis, J.E. Blackmon, and S. Bober. "Sexual Dysfunction in Young Adult Survivors of Childhood Cancer." *Pediatric Blood & Cancer* 63, no. 9 (September 2016): 1,622–28.

Reinman, L., H.L. Coons, J. Sopfe, and R. Casey. "Psychosexual Care of Adolescent and Young Adult (AYA) Cancer Survivors." *Children (Basel)* 8, no. 11 (November 16, 2021): 1,058.

Stanton, A.M., A.B. Handy, and C.M. Meston. "Sexual Function in Adolescents and Young Adults Diagnosed with Cancer: A Systematic Review." *Journal of Cancer Survivorship* 12, no. 1 (February 2018): 47–63.

Zhou, E.S., N.N. Frederick, and S.L. Bober. "Hormonal Changes and Sexual Dysfunction." *Medical Clinics of North America* 101, no. 6 (November 2017): 1,135–50.

Zhou, E.S., S.J. Falk, and S.L. Bober. "Managing Premature Menopause and Sexual Dysfunction." *Current Opinion in Supportive and Palliative Care* 9, no. 3 (September 2015): 294–300.

Chapter 10

Johnston, E.E., and A.R. Rosenberg. "Palliative Care in Adolescents and Young Adults with Cancer." *Journal of Clinical Oncology* 42, no. 6 (February 20, 2024): 755–63.

Mack, J.W., et al. "Discussions about Goals of Care and Advance Care Planning among Adolescents and Young Adults with Cancer Approaching the End of Life." *Journal of Clinical Oncology* 41, no. 30 (October 20, 2023): 4,739–46.

Mack, J.W., et al. "Quality of End-of-Life Care among Adolescents and Young Adults with Cancer." *Journal of Clinical Oncology* 42, no. 6 (February 20, 2024): 621–29.

Perez, G.K., et al. "Taboo Topics in Adolescent and Young Adult Oncology: Strategies for Managing Challenging but Important Conversations Central to Adolescent and Young Adult Cancer Survivorship." *American Society of Clinical Oncology Educational Book* 40 (March 2020): 1–15.

Resources

General Cancer Resources

American Cancer Society
www.cancer.org
Offers comprehensive support, education, and advocacy for cancer patients and their families.

American Childhood Cancer Organization
www.acco.org
Works to shape public policy, raise awareness, and provide resources for children with cancer and their families.

American Society of Clinical Oncology
www.asco.org
Organization for physicians and oncology professionals caring for people with cancer.

The Dear Jack Foundation
www.dearjackfoundation.org
Provides a range of programming to improve quality of life.

Leukemia & Lymphoma Society
www.lls.org
Supports blood cancer patients with education, financial aid, and advocacy, including Spanish-language resources.

National Cancer Institute
www.cancer.gov
A leading resource for cancer research, treatment information, and clinical trials.

Susan G. Komen
www.komen.org
Leading national resource on breast cancer.

Teenage Cancer Trust
www.teenagecancertrust.org
United Kingdom–based group offering resources and support.

Financial and Legal Assistance

Allyson Whitney Foundation
www.allysonwhitney.org
Provides financial assistance (including for fertility) through "Life Interrupted Grants" to young adults with rare cancers.

Cancer Financial Assistance Coalition
www.cancerfac.org
A group of organizations helping cancer patients with their finances.

Expect Miracles Foundation's SAMFund
www.expectmiraclesfoundation.org/samfund

Provides general financial assistance and family-building grants to support young adult cancer survivors.

Family Reach
www.familyreach.org
Delivers financial support and education to families struggling with the financial burden of cancer treatment.

Patient Advocate Foundation
www.patientadvocate.org
Provides case management and financial aid to patients, including resources in Spanish.

Academic and Career (Including Scholarships and Grants)

Cancer and Careers
www.cancerandcareers.org
Helps people with cancer thrive in their workplaces.

Cancer for College
https://cancerforcollege.org
Provides scholarships and debt relief for cancer survivors.

Michael A. Hunter Memorial Scholarship
www.oc-cf.org/scholarships/available-scholarships
Offers scholarships for leukemia/lymphoma patients or survivors, or children of nonsurviving leukemia/lymphoma patients.

National Grace Foundation
www.graceamerica.org
Helps send pediatric cancer survivors to college.

The Ruth Cheatham Foundation
www.ruthcheathamfoundation.org
Supports education opportunities for teens and young adults with cancer.

Fertility Resources

Alliance for Fertility Preservation
www.allianceforfertilitypreservation.org
Provides professional advice on fertility preservation.

Allyson Whitney Foundation
www.allysonwhitney.org
Provides financial assistance (including for fertility) through "Life Interrupted Grants" to young adults with rare cancers.

Expect Miracles Foundation's SAMFund
www.expectmiraclesfoundation.org/samfund
Provides general financial assistance and family-building grants to support young adult cancer survivors.

Resolve: The National Infertility Association
www.resolve.org
Offers resources and support for family building.

Save My Fertility
www.savemyfertility.org
Resources for preserving fertility before and during cancer treatment.

Team Maggie's Dream
www.teammaggiesdream.org
Offers financial support for fertility preservation during cancer treatment.

Tinina Q. Cade Foundation
https://cadefoundation.org
Offers resources and grants for cancer patients managing fertility challenges.

Verna's Purse
https://reprotech.com/vernas-purse
Helps cancer patients pay for fertility-preservation services.

Worth the Wait
www.worththewaitcharity.com
Provides fertility and adoption grants for cancer survivors.

Legal Assistance

Disability Rights Legal Center
https://thedrlc.org/cancer
Answers legal questions for people with cancer. Also offers a legal handbook in English and Spanish.

Just Great Lawyers: Legal Resources for Cancer Patients
www.justgreatlawyers.com/legal-resources-for-cancer-patients
Lists a collection of resources for cancer patients.

Triage Cancer
www.triagecancer.org
Provides free education on legal issues related to cancer.

Lodging Assistance

American Cancer Society's Hope Lodge and Extended Stay America Partnership
www.cancer.org
Provides lodging options for cancer patients.

Open Arms Foundation
https://openarmsfoundation.networkforgood.com
Provides lodging options for medical patients.

Resources to Help with Physical Changes

Chemocessories
https://chemocessories.org
Organization that donates scarves and jewelry to people going through treatment.

EBeauty Community for Cancer Support
https://ebeauty.com
Offers free wigs to rebuild confidence during cancer treatment.

Heavenly Hats
www.heavenlyhats.org
Distributes hats to those with hair loss.

Hope Scarves
www.hopescarves.org
Supplies scarves to cancer patients.

Look Good Feel Better
www.lookgoodfeelbetter.org
Offers guidance on beauty techniques to address appearance-related side effects of cancer.

Verma Foundation
www.vermafoundation.org
Provides free, high-quality cap wigs.

Wigs and Wishes
www.wigsandwishes.org
Provides wigs to those facing cancer.

Keeping People Informed

CaringBridge
www.caringbridge.org
A trusted communication platform
where people can share updates and
find community.

ianacare
www.ianacare.com
Platform for caregivers to share
information.

Lotsa Helping Hands
www.lotsahelpinghands.com
Provides a way to organize meals and
support for someone in need.

National Support Programs and Support Groups for Early Adulthood Cancer

Cactus Cancer Society
www.cactuscancer.org
Offers free creative and expression-
based online programs for young
adult patients and survivors.

**Cancer Care Online Support
Groups**
https://cancercare.org/support_
groups/147-young_adults_with_
cancer_support_group
A free fifteen-week online support
group for young adults (ages twenty
to thirty-nine) currently receiving
treatment.

**Cancer Support Community and
Gilda's Club**
www.cancersupportcommunity.org

Offers free support, education, and
community and a toll-free helpline
for anyone impacted by cancer,
including patients and caregivers.

Dempsey Center
www.dempseycenter.org
Provides free personalized care,
including counseling, nutrition
information, and integrative therapies,
for cancer patients and families.

Elephants and Tea
www.elephantsandtea.org
A magazine and community for
young adult cancer patients,
survivors, and caregivers. Offers
events and support groups.

Stupid Cancer
www.stupidcancer.org
Provides resources, events, and a
community to help young adults
navigate cancer and survivorship.

Resources for Patients with Children

Bright Spot Network
www.brightspotnetwork.org
Provides support groups, financial
grants, and resources for parents with
cancer and their young children.

Camp Kesem
www.kesem.org
Offers free summer camps and
programs for children coping with a
parent's cancer.

The Children's Treehouse Foundation
www.childrenstreehousefdn.org
Offers programming to help children develop coping strategies when a parent is diagnosed with cancer.

Hope Connections
www.hopeconnectionsforcancer.org
Professionally led programs for families to address the emotional and physical impacts of cancer.

Pickles Group
www.picklesgroup.org
Free peer-to-peer support for kids and teens whose parents or guardians have cancer.

Wonders and Worries
www.wondersandworries.org
Professional support for children and teens during a parent's serious illness or injury.

Books

Cancer in Our Family by the American Cancer Society

Raising an Emotionally Healthy Child When a Parent Is Sick by Paula K. Rauch, MD, and Anna C. Muriel, MD, MPH

Someone I Love Is Sick: Helping Very Young Children Cope with Cancer in the Family by Kathleen McCue, MA, LSW, CCLS

When a Parent Has Cancer: A Guide to Caring for Your Children by Wendy S. Harpham, MD

Sexual Health

American Association of Sexuality Educators, Counselors and Therapists
www.aasect.org
Provides a list of practitioners in your area.

American Cancer Society: Sexual Side Effects
www.cancer.org/cancer/managing-cancer/side-effects/sexual-side-effects.html
Comprehensive information on how cancer and its treatments can impact sexual health, intimacy, and body image.

Living Beyond Breast Cancer: Sex & Intimacy
www.lbbc.org/about-breast-cancer/family-relationships/sex-and-intimacy
Guidance on managing intimacy, body image, and sexual health after breast cancer.

National LGBT Cancer Network
www.cancer-network.org
Provides support and resources for LGBTQ+ individuals affected by cancer, including peer support groups.

Society for Sex Therapy and Research
https://sstarnet.org/find-therapist
Locate qualified therapists specializing in sex therapy, sexual health, and relationships.

Care Planning for Advancing Cancer

Five Wishes
www.fivewishes.org
A simple, user-friendly advance directive helping adults and adolescents communicate their care preferences and end-of-life wishes.

Books

A Beginner's Guide to the End by BJ Miller, MD, and Shoshana Berger

Being Mortal by Atul Gawande, MD

When Breath Becomes Air by Paul Kalanithi, MD

Voicing My Choices (available at https://ccr.cancer.gov).

Integrative Medicine

These resources include information on meditation, activity/exercise options, nutrition, therapeutic massage, acupuncture, and expressive arts.

Livestrong at the YMCA
https://livestrong.org/how-we-help/livestrong-at-the-ymca
A twelve-week physical activity program for adult cancer survivors, focusing on regaining strength, improving fitness, and enhancing quality of life.

Memorial Sloan Kettering Cancer Center About Herbs App
www.mskcc.org/cancer-care/diagnosis-treatment/symptom-management/integrative-medicine/herbs/about-herbs
A mobile app offering evidence-based information on herbs, botanicals, and supplements for patients and healthcare providers.

Osher Collaborative for Integrative Medicine
www.oshercollaborative.org
A group of several academic centers that study, teach, and practice integrative health.

Insomnia

American Academy of Sleep Medicine
www.aasm.org
Provides detailed guidelines and resources on diagnosing and managing insomnia.

National Heart, Lung, and Blood Institute: *Your Guide to Healthy Sleep*
www.nhlbi.nih.gov/resources/your-guide-healthy-sleep
An e-booklet providing science-based insights into sleep health.

National Sleep Foundation
www.sleepfoundation.org
A trusted resource offering expert sleep advice, product reviews, and evidence-based health content.

INDEX

Acceptance and commitment therapy (ACT), 164, 169

Acute lymphocytic leukemia (ALL), 37

Acute myeloid leukemia (AML), 37, 99–100

Alcohol use, 31, 66, 69, 131, 153, 207

American Cancer Society (ACS), 11, 18–20, 37, 121

American Society for Reproductive Medicine (ASRM), 44

American Society of Clinical Oncology (ASCO), 44

Barr, Mark, 182

Body image, 75, 89, 110, 182, 198–99, 208–10

Brain tumor, 16, 26, 37, 153

Breast cancer, 18–19, 25, 39, 53–54, 60, 66, 72–73, 88–89, 102, 130, 149–50, 158, 162, 183, 193, 197, 206–7, 215

Breitbart, William S., 226

Cancer diagnosis
delayed diagnoses, 21–24, 29
explaining to children, 56–61, 68, 84
late diagnoses, 21–24, 29
missed diagnoses, 21–24, 29
overlooking health issues, 21–23
reactions to, 11–12, 16–17, 31–39, 53–54
risky behaviors and, 23–24, 130
second opinions on, 38, 42, 52, 215
sharing news about, 37, 53–68, 113–18

Cancer patients. *See also* Patient experiences
older patients, 12, 17, 25, 40–41
pediatric patients, 12, 17, 25–26, 29, 41
young adult patients, 11–12, 15–29, 39–42

Cancer recurrence, 25, 101, 132, 153, 174–78, 214–20, 228, 234. *See also* Relapse

Cancer screening guidelines, 19–21

Cancer treatments. *See also* Surgery
advances in, 20–21
chemotherapy, 20, 44, 46, 77–95, 98, 154, 181–86
coping with, 69–170
cost of, 119–21
fatigue from, 77–78, 80–81, 90–95, 97–98, 181–86
fertility concerns and, 43–52, 180, 195–96
financial concerns and, 23, 101, 114, 119–21, 223
guidelines for, 40, 44, 48
immunotherapies, 39, 44, 46, 71, 97–98, 154, 218, 222
integrative therapies, 20, 66–67, 93–96, 150, 185–87, 214
life changes and, 99–123, 149–69, 171–92, 213–34
nutrition and, 66, 87–92, 134, 181
outcomes of, 20–21, 71–72, 177
post-treatment life, 149–69, 171–92
psychotherapy and, 149–69
quality of life and, 20, 46, 65–66, 90, 117–20, 126–27, 178, 217–18, 230–33
radiation therapy, 44–47, 51–54, 64–65, 70–71, 75–77
side effects from, 20, 46, 73–98, 132–33, 154, 181–86, 193–211
targeted therapies, 44, 46, 71, 97, 196, 213–15, 218, 222

Cancers. *See also specific types*
chronic cancer, 37, 179, 213–34
coping with, 15–29, 31–123, 125–69, 171–211, 213–36
early days of, 31–52
early onset cancer, 11–21, 27–29, 48, 161, 168–69, 206

increases in, 11–12, 18–20, 29
screening for, 19–21
sharing news about, 37, 53–68, 113–18
stress and, 129–38, 141–48
Care team, 13, 26, 40–44, 60–68, 70–79, 121, 158, 214–34. *See also* Clinical team; Medical team; Oncology team
CaringBridge, 61
Checkups, regular, 22–23, 69, 102, 110
Chemotherapy
  "chemo brain," 93–95, 185–86
  cognitive changes, 93–95, 185–86
  description of, 20, 44, 46, 77–89
  fatigue and, 80–81, 90–95, 97–98, 181–86
  hair loss and, 20, 81–85
  nausea and, 20, 80–81, 85–87
  nutritional challenges and, 87–92
  prepping for, 78–79
  side effects from, 20, 46, 78–95, 98, 154, 181–86
  weight changes and, 20, 89, 181
Chronic cancer, 37, 179, 213–34
Chronic lymphocytic leukemia (CLL), 37
Clinical team, 38–44, 54–55, 63–68, 78–79, 97, 111–12, 119, 151, 223. *See also* Care team; Medical team; Oncology team
Clinical trials, 37–38, 41, 215, 230, 232
Cognitive behavioral therapy (CBT), 163–64, 169, 184
Colon/colorectal cancer, 18–21, 25, 39–42, 46–47, 74, 88, 125–26, 197, 213–14
Coping
  with cancer, 15–29, 31–123, 125–69, 171–211, 213–36
  with cancer treatment, 69–170
  with chronic cancer, 37, 179, 213–34
  with emotional changes, 58, 99–123, 150, 153–57
  with life changes, 99–123, 149–69, 171–92, 213–34

with post-treatment life, 149–69, 171–92

Dana-Farber Cancer Institute, 11, 61, 65, 80, 99–100, 156, 226
Diagnosis. *See* Cancer diagnosis
Diet/nutrition, 38, 66, 69–70, 87–92, 134–35, 138, 181
"Dr. Google," 37–38, 52
Doctors, finding, 39–43. *See also* Medical team; Oncology team

Emotions
  cancer diagnosis and, 11–12, 16–17, 31–39, 53–54
  emotional changes, 58, 99–123, 150, 153–57
  fight-or-flight response, 35–36, 70, 128, 133, 177
  mood changes, 27, 60, 93, 100, 138–41, 147, 152–68, 177, 191, 201–2, 209
  toxic positivity and, 104–9, 122–23, 187–88
European Society for Medical Oncology, 44
Exercise, 111, 125–26, 135–38, 142, 146–50, 177, 181, 184–87, 221

Facebook, 55, 115
Family and Medical Leave Act (FMLA), 111
Family support, 26–28, 51, 111–23
Fear of cancer recurrence (FCR), 174–78, 228
Fear of missing out (FOMO), 115–16
Feelings of being overwhelmed, 11–12, 16–17, 31–39, 51–55. *See also* Emotions
Fertility
  concerns about, 43–52, 180, 195–96
  female fertility preservation, 50–51
  fertility-preservation options, 44, 47–51
  male fertility preservation, 50
  oncofertility, 44–49

Fight-or-flight response, 35–36, 70, 128, 133, 177

Financial concerns, 23, 101, 114, 119–21, 223

Five Wishes, 231

Friends
 reestablishing friendships, 187–90, 226–28
 social isolation and, 105, 116–19, 161–62, 167, 169, 226–27
 support from, 26–27, 51, 113–23

Gastrointestinal cancers, 41, 46

Gland tumors, 19, 153

Google, 37–38, 52

Guidelines, screening, 19–21

Guidelines, treatment, 40, 44, 48

Harvard Medical School, 11, 65, 156

Head/neck cancer, 66, 69–75, 88, 101, 197

Health. *See also* Mental health; Sexual health
 focusing on, 28–29, 125–48, 180–92
 overlooking health issues, 21–23
 risky behaviors and, 23–24, 130
 self-care and, 28–29, 125–48, 180–92
 well-being and, 28–29, 82, 125–48, 168, 178–81, 207–11, 226–36

Hobbies/activities, 117, 138–42. *See also* Exercise

Hodgkin lymphoma, 32, 215

Immunotherapies, 39, 44, 46, 71, 97–98, 154, 218, 222

Instagram, 55, 115

Integrative therapies, 20, 66–67, 93–96, 150, 185–87, 214

Leukemia, 37, 40, 51, 60, 64, 89, 99–100, 121, 215

Life changes
 autonomy and, 111–13, 123
 chronic cancer and, 37, 179, 213–34
 coping with, 99–123, 149–69, 171–92, 213–34

emotional changes, 58, 99–123, 150, 153–57

life purpose and, 145, 164–67, 226–28, 234–36

post-treatment life, 149–69, 171–92

quality of life, 20, 46, 65–66, 90, 117–20, 126–27, 178, 217–18, 230–33

uncertainty and, 33–37, 62, 121–22, 128–31, 173–74, 219–21

Livestrong, 182

Lotsa Helping Hands, 61

Lung cancer, 16, 25, 39, 65–66, 74, 213–14, 218

Lymphoma, 32, 37, 60, 121, 171, 215

Medical team, 20, 37–52, 55–96, 196–204, 222–23. *See also* Care team; Clinical team; Oncology team

Memorial Sloan Kettering Cancer Center, 209, 226

Memories Live, 232

Mental health
 mental health professionals, 58, 66, 72–73, 96, 149–69, 178–79, 224–25, 229, 231–32
 relationships and, 116–19
 self-care and, 125–48, 180–92
 severe symptoms and, 58, 93–95, 151–54, 163–64, 186–87
 social isolation and, 105, 116–19, 161–62, 167, 169, 226–27
 stress and, 119–22, 125–48, 161–64, 172–78, 183–87, 223–30
 well-being and, 82, 125–48, 168, 178–81, 207–11, 226–36

Metastatic cancer, 16, 47, 174, 213–19, 234

Metastatic, recurrent, or relapsed (MRR) cancer, 217–30, 234

Mindfulness/meditation, 96, 132, 138–39, 143–49, 166, 177, 185–87, 214

Mortality, grasping, 24, 121–22, 128, 220–21, 234

Muscles, 75, 89, 97, 181–82, 198, 204–5

National Cancer Institute (NCI), 17, 21, 37–38, 40, 44, 47
National Comprehensive Cancer Network (NCCN), 40
National Institute of Mental Health (NIMH), 126
National Institutes of Health (NIH), 44, 47
New normal, 172, 178–81, 185–87, 198–99, 211

Oncofertility, 44–49. *See also* Fertility
Oncologists, finding, 39–43. *See also* Oncology team
Oncology spaces, 24–26, 29
Oncology team, 37–52, 55–96, 117, 140, 157–62, 171–85, 196–204, 209–10, 214–34

Pain management, 20, 146, 157–58, 168, 222, 230–31
Palliative care team, 65–66, 77, 158, 214, 217, 222, 230–31. *See also* Care team
Pancreatic cancer, 25
Partner/spouse support, 26–28, 51, 111–13, 206–11
Patient experiences
    Aaidaliz, 156
    Amber, 59
    Ashlyn, 179
    Bethany, 236
    Brook, 171–72, 174
    Chloe, 193–94, 201
    Christy, 207–8
    Cindy, 149–50
    Colleen, 118
    Daniella, 15–19
    Darren, 144–45
    Deja, 42
    Glenn, 213–14
    Greg, 31–33, 52
    Jeremy, 25
    Jessica, 34
    John, 61
    Keisha, 99–100
    Madison, 107
    Maria, 53–55
    Matt, 69–73
    Molly, 125–27
    Orsolya, 136
    Sarah, 188
    Shirley, 22–23
    Valerie, 218
Pediatric oncology patients, 12, 17, 25–26, 29, 41
Pets, benefits of, 139, 146–48
Post-treatment life, 149–69, 171–92
Pozo-Kaderman, Cristina, 11–13
Prostate cancer, 47
Psychopharmacology, 167–68
Psychotherapy. *See also* Mental health
    benefits of, 149–69, 194–95, 211, 219–26
    finding therapists, 155–56
    group therapy options, 161–63, 169
    importance of, 149–69
    process of, 159–61
    psychopharmacology, 167–68
    severe symptoms and, 151–54, 163–64, 186–87
    specific approaches, 163–64, 169, 184
Purpose/meaning, 145, 164–67, 226–28, 234–36

Radiation therapy, 44–47, 51–54, 64–65, 70–71, 75–77
Recreational drug use, 66–69, 110, 130, 152–53, 157–58, 222
Relapse, 214–15, 217–30, 234. *See also* Cancer recurrence
Relaxation techniques, 93–96, 132, 136–49, 164–67, 177, 185–87, 208, 214
Resources, 245–50

Sarcoma, 18, 37, 40, 75
Screening guidelines, 19–21
Second opinions, 38, 42, 52, 215
Self-care, 28–29, 125–48, 180–92. *See also* Relaxation techniques
Sexual health
    changes in, 193–211
    contraception and, 196–97
    dating and, 206–8, 211

enhancing intimacy, 207–11
female-related issues, 193–94,
  201–6, 209
male-related issues, 199–201
pregnancy and, 196–97
Sharing news/updates, 37, 53–68, 113–18
Side effects
  from cancer treatments, 20, 46,
    73–98, 132–33, 154, 181–86,
    193–211
  from chemotherapy, 20, 46, 78–95,
    97–98, 154, 181–86
  fatigue, 77–78, 80–81, 90–95,
    97–98, 181–86
  hair loss, 20, 81–85
  from immunotherapies, 46,
    97–98, 154
  nausea, 20, 80–81, 85–87, 95–97,
    132–33
  post-treatment effects, 181–82
  from radiation therapy, 46–47,
    75–77
  from surgery, 47, 73–75
  from targeted therapies, 46, 97, 196
  weight changes, 20, 89, 181
Sleep issues, 90–95, 148–54, 181–86,
  198–204, 231–33
Sleep requirements, 136
Sloan Kettering Cancer Center, 209,
  226
Social isolation, 105, 116–19, 161–62,
  167, 169, 226–27
Social media, 37, 55, 62–63, 113–18,
  142
Spirituality/faith, 101–6, 127, 132,
  138–41, 165–66, 178, 183, 226–27,
  231
Stress management, 119–22, 125–48,
  161–64, 172–78, 183–87, 223–30. *See
  also* Relaxation techniques
Supplements/herbs, 54, 66–68, 87,
  96, 209
Support
  from family, 26–28, 51, 111–23
  from friends, 26–27, 51, 113–23
  from partner/spouse, 26–28, 51,
    111–13, 206–11

professional support, 45, 150–52,
  229–30
support groups, 61, 99–100, 114,
  118–19, 161–63, 169, 192, 230–34
Surgery
  description of, 71–75
  head/neck surgery, 66, 69–75, 101
  impact of, 47, 73–75
  lumpectomy, 53–54, 72
  mastectomy, 53–54, 66, 72, 193
  reconstructive surgeries, 53–54,
    66, 72–73, 158, 193
  surgical oncologists, 64, 66
  testicular surgery, 47, 73
Survivor's guilt, 190–92

Targeted therapies, 44, 46, 71, 97,
  196, 213–15, 218, 222
Testicular cancer, 47, 73, 75, 215
TikTok, 140
Toxic positivity, 104–9, 122–23, 187–88
Treatments. *See* Cancer treatments

Updates, sharing, 53–68, 113–18

Vitamins, 66–68. *See also*
  Supplements/herbs
"Voicing My Choices," 231

Well-being, 28–29, 82, 125–48, 168,
  178–81, 207–11, 226–36
Whitmore, Jamie, 182
Wisnia, Saul, 12
Woodruff, Teresa, 44

Young Adult Program (YAP), 11,
  99–100
Young adults. *See also* Patient
  experiences
  differences for, 15–29, 39–42
  feeling out of place, 24–26, 29
  increases in cancer for, 11–12,
    18–20, 29
YouTube, 37, 140

Zoom, 116, 127, 132

About the Authors

Cristina Pozo-Kaderman, PhD, is a senior psychologist, director of Interprofessional Education, and director of the Young Adult Program (YAP) in the Department of Supportive Oncology at Dana-Farber Cancer Institute with a faculty appointment at Harvard Medical School. Dr. Pozo-Kaderman obtained her doctorate in clinical psychology from the University of Miami. She completed her internship at Cornell Medical College, Payne Whitney Clinic, and her fellowship in psycho-oncology at Memorial Sloan Kettering Cancer Center. For more than thirty years, she has worked in the field of psychosocial oncology with young adults, mentoring trainees as well as serving on numerous professional and community organizations.

Saul Wisnia has been senior publications editor-writer at Dana-Farber Cancer Institute since 1999. He is a former sports and news correspondent at *The Washington Post* and feature reporter at the *Boston Herald*. His articles have also appeared in *The Boston Globe*, *Sports Illustrated*, and many other publications. Wisnia is the author or coauthor of numerous books, including the *Library Journal*–starred *Spinal Cord Injury and the Family* and *The Jimmy Fund of Dana-Farber Cancer Institute*. He lives with his wife and dog just outside Boston.